Atlas of Fetal Sectional Anatomy

G. Isaacson   M.C. Mintz   E.S. Crelin

Atlas of Fetal Sectional Anatomy

With Ultrasound and Magnetic Resonance Imaging

With 278 Illustrations

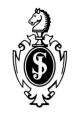

Springer-Verlag
New York Berlin Heidelberg Tokyo

Glenn Isaacson, M.D.
Attending Surgeon, Pennsylvania Hospital, Eighth and Spruce Streets, Philadelphia,
Pennsylvania 19104, U.S.A.

Marshall C. Mintz, M.D.
Assistant Professor, Department of Radiology, Hospital of the University of
Pennsylvania, 3400 Spruce Street, Philadelphia, Pennsylvania 19104, U.S.A.

Edmund S. Crelin, Ph.D., DSc.
Professor of Anatomy, Department of Surgery, Yale University School of Medicine, 333 Cedar Street, New Haven, Connecticut 06510, U.S.A.

Library of Congress Cataloging in Publication Data
Isaacson, G. (Glenn)
    Atlas of fetal sectional anatomy with ultrasound and magnetic resonance imaging.
    Includes index.
    1. Ultrasonics in obstetrics.   2. Fetus—Anatomy.
I. Mintz, M. C. (Marshall C.)   II. Crelin, Edmund S.,
1923–   .   III. Title. [DNLM: 1. Fetus—anatomy &
histology—atlases.   2. Ultrasonic Diagnosis—atlases.
WQ 17 I73a]
RG527.5.U48I83   1986   618.3′207543   85-27901

Ultrasound on p. 9 and gross figure and ultrasound on p. 23 from Isaacson, G., Mintz,
M.C: Ultrasound Visualization of the Inner Ear Before Birth. J Ultrasound Med., In Press.
Reprinted with permission from W. B. Saunders Co.

Typeset by David E. Seham Associates Inc., Metuchen, New Jersey.
Printed and bound by Halliday Lithograph, West Hanover, Massachusetts.
Printed in the United States of America.

9 8 7 6 5 4 3 2 1

ISBN 0-387-96248-4 Springer-Verlag New York Berlin Heidelberg
ISBN 3-540-96248-4 Springer-Verlag Berlin Heidelberg New York

Preface

The fetal period of human growth and development has become an area of intense study in recent years, due in large part to the development of diagnostic ultrasound. More than 2,000 articles have been published in the last five years describing anatomy and pathology *in utero,* as reflected in sonographic images. Yet, no standard reference exists to correlate these images with fetal gross anatomy and attempts to draw parallels from adult structure have often led to false assumptions. The dictum "the newborn is not a miniature adult" is all the more valid for the fetus.

This text aims to provide a comprehensive reference for normal sectional anatomy correlated with *in utero* ultrasound images. In addition, magnetic resonance images of therapeutically aborted or stillborn fetuses are paired with similar gross sections to serve as a foundation upon which current *in vivo* studies may build. Lastly, a miscellaneous section illustrates several anatomic points useful in the understanding of fetal anatomy. These points include the changing anatomy of the fetal brain during gestation and the anatomy of the meninges, the fetal heart, and ductus venosus.

It is our hope that this atlas will provide a clear picture of fetal anatomy, rectify some of the confusion which exists in antenatal diagnosis, and stimulate further interest in fetal development.

October, 1985

Glenn Isaacson
Marshall C. Mintz
Edmund S. Crelin

Acknowledgments

We wish to acknowledge the support, guidance and inspiration of John Decker of the Department of Pathology at Pennsylvania Hospital, Richard Ochs at Temple University School of Medicine and G. J. Walker Smith at Yale University School of Medicine.

Special thanks to Harold Kundel, Peter Joseph, and Debbie DeSimone, Department of Radiology, Hospital of the University of Pennsylvania for their invaluable assistance with the MR images. The ultrasound technicians at the Hospital of the University of Pennsylvania also deserve mention for their help with the sonographic images.

June Connolly deserves praise for her tireless work in the preparation of the manuscript.

This research was supported in part by Public Health Service Biomedical Research Support Grant #2S07RR05590 from the Pennsylvania Hospital Research Review Committee and the Crippled Children's Aid Society of New Haven, Connecticut.

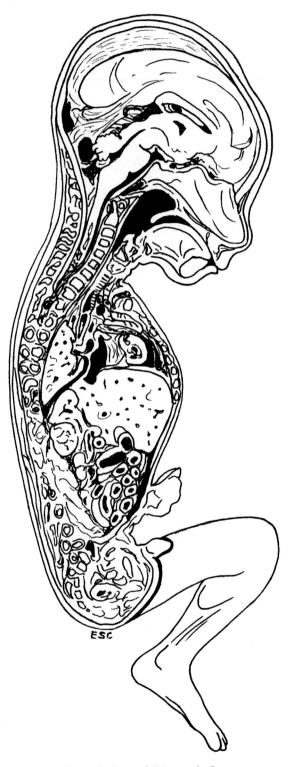

Actual size of 20 week fetus.

Contents

Methods and Materials xi

Fetal Head and Neck 1

  1 Sagittal Sections 1
  2 Coronal Sections 13
  3 Axial Sections 31

Fetal Thorax and Abdomen 57

  1 Axial Sections 57
     Male Thorax and Abdomen 57
     Male Pelvis 83
     Female Pelvis 93
  2 Sagittal Sections 103
  3 Coronal Sections 119

Fetal Limbs 127

Special Studies 149

  1 Fetal Brain Development 149
     Cortical Development 150
     Ventricular Development 154
     Dural Structures 158
  2 Anatomy of the Ductus Venosus 159
  3 Fetal Heart 163

Index 175

Methods and Materials

Gross Sections

Anatomic sections were made using fetal cadavers which were the products of second trimester therapeutic abortions. The third trimester specimens used were spontaneous abortuses, but were grossly free of structural abnormalities.

Fetal head specimens were fixed by cannulating the common carotid artery and perfusing the head overnight with a 10% formalin–5% acetic acid mixture followed by injection of the subarachnoid space and immersion in the same fixative for one week. The fixed fetal heads were then frozen at $-4°C$ for 24 hours and sectioned on a band saw. Sawing artifact was minimized by wiping the still frozen sections with a gloved finger in a rapid stream of tap water. Transverse sections of the cranium were cut at 10° above Reid's baseline: Those through the face and neck were cut perpendicular to the fetal long axis. Sections were thawed prior to photographing them.

Specimens used for thorax, abdomen and pelvis sections were fixed by immersion in 10% formalin in fetal position. Sections were cut at room temperature using a long, smooth knife perpendicular to the fetal spine.

Photographs were made using an Olympus OM-1, single lens reflex, 35 mm camera with 50 mm macro lens and Kodak Technical Pan film. The specimens were illuminated by four tungsten lamps, each one meter from the subject with polarizing filters between the lamps and the specimens and a crossed polarizing filter mounted on the camera lens. The specimens were photographed following the radiographic conventions of viewing transverse sections from caudal to cranial and coronal sections from ventral to dorsal.

Sections were labelled in accordance with the Nomina Anatomica, using anglicized versions of the Latin designation when possible and including common eponyms in parentheses.

Ultrasound and Magnetic Resonance Images

Sonographic images were generated during routine obstetrical examinations upon fetuses of approximately 20 weeks gestation. GE RT 3000 (3.5 MHz linear array), Diasonics DRF 400 and RA-1 (3.5 MHz sector scanner), and Acuson 128 (3.5 MHz linear array) units were used.

Magnetic resonance examinations were performed upon therapeutically aborted or stillborn fetuses of 21–24 weeks gestational age. A 1.5 Tesla superconducting magnetic resonance imager with a 6.5 inch transmitter coil and a 3 or 4 inch receiver coil was used. The magnification factor is 1.7–2.9 and the pixel size is 0.4–0.8 mm. The matrix is 128 x 128. Inversion recovery axial images with repetition time (TR) = 2000 msec and time to inversion (TI) = 1000 msec, as well as spin echo T_2 weighted axial images with (TR) = 2000 msec and echo time (TE) = 150 msec were obtained. The slice thickness of these images is 2–3 mm. From these techniques, the image which best illustrated anatomic detail was selected at each section level. Coronal and sagittal images are all T_2 weighted with a slice thickness of 3 mm.

Fetal Head and Neck

SECTION 1

Sagittal Sections

34 Week Fetus

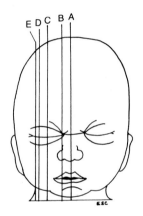

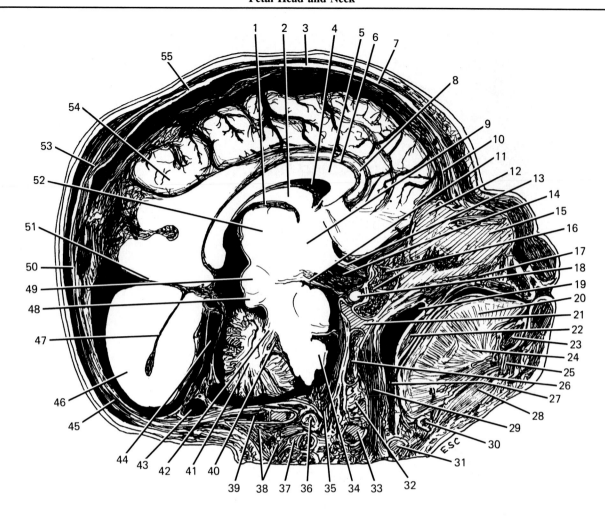

1–Choroid fissure
2–Fornix
3–Anterior fonticulus (fontanelle)
4–Left lateral ventricle
5–Corpus callosum
6–Sulcus of corpus callosum
7–Frontal suture
8–Cingulate gyrus
9–Hypothalamus
10–Frontal bone
11–Oculomotor nerve
12–Crista galli
13–Left optic nerve
14–Chiasmatic cistern
15–Nasal septum
16–Body of sphenoid bone
17–Hard palate
18–Pituitary gland
19–Nasopharynx
20–Tongue

21–Spheno-occipital synchondrosis
22–Soft palate
23–Left 1st deciduous incisor tooth
24–Genioglossus muscle
25–Body of mandible
26–Basilar part of occipital bone
27–Oropharynx
28–Geniohyoid muscle
29–Longus colli muscle
30–Hyoid bone
31–Arytenoid cartilage
32–Atlanto-occipital joint
33–Axis
34–Olive
35–Foramen magnum
36–Posterior arch of atlas
37–Spinous process of axis
38–Deep craniovertebral muscles
39–Lateral part of occipital bone
40–4th ventricle

41–Cerebellar hemisphere
42–Superior cerebellar peduncle
43–Transverse sinus
44–Straight sinus
45–Squamous part of occipital bone
46–Occipital lobe
47–Calcarine fissure
48–Inferior colliculus
49–Superior colliculus
50–Posterior fonticulus (fontanelle)
51–Parieto-occipital sulcus
52–Thalamus
53–Parietal bone
54–Parietal lobe
55–Sagittal suture
56–Pons
57–Midbrain
58–Frontal lobe
59–Vermis

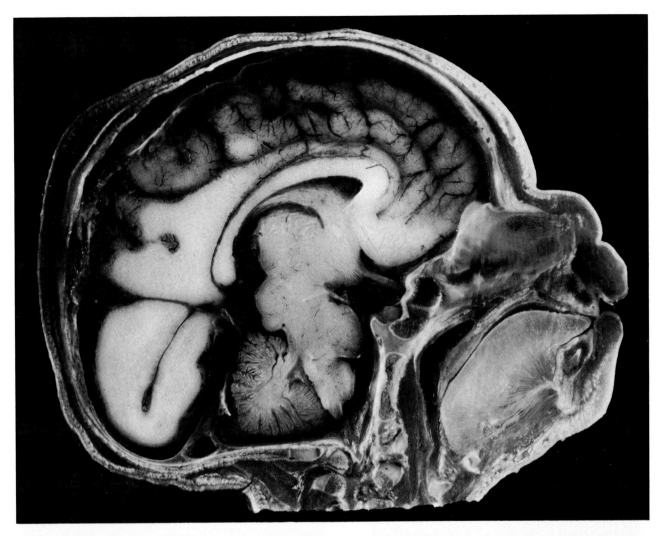

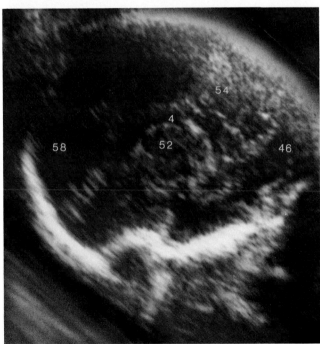

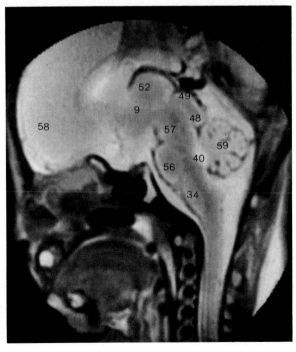

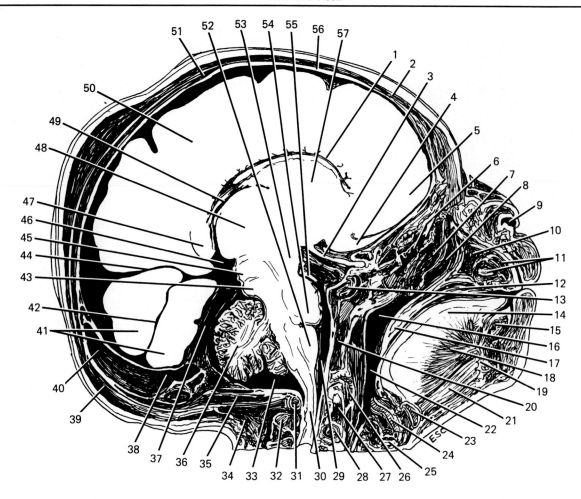

1–Sulcus of corpus callosum
2–Frontal bone
3–Right optic nerve
4–Olfactory tract
5–Frontal lobe
6–Ethmoid sinuses
7–Inferior nasal concha
8–Inferior nasal meatus
9–Naris
10–Maxilla
11–1st and 2nd right deciduous incisor
teeth
12–Hard palate
13–Pituitary gland
14–Tongue
15–Right 1st deciduous incisor tooth
16–Nasopharynx
17–Soft palate
18–Genioglossus muscle
19–Mandible
20–Basilar part of occipital bone

21–Geniohyoid muscle
22–Oropharynx
23–Hyoid bone
24–Epiglottis
25–Vocal fold (cord)
26–Anterior arch of atlas
27–Dens of axis
28–C₃ vertebra
29–Basilar artery
30–Spinal medulla (cord)
31–Posterior arch of atlas
32–Spinous process of axis
33–Cerebellomedullaris cistern
(cisterna magna)
34–Deep craniovertebral muscles
35–Lateral part of occipital bone
36–Cerebellum
37–Straight sinus
38–Confluence of sinuses
39–Squamous part of occipital bone
40–Superior sagittal sinus

41–Occipital lobe
42–Calcarine sulcus
43–Inferior colliculus
44–Parieto-occipital sulcus
45–Superior colliculus
46–Cistern of great cerebral vein
(ambiens)
47–Splenium of corpus callosum
48–Thalamus
49–Choroid fissure
50–Parietal lobe
51–Parietal bone
52–Olive
53–Cerebral peduncle
54–Pons
55–Oculomotor nerve
56–Anterior fonticulus (fontanelle)
57–Septum pellucidum
58–Eyeball

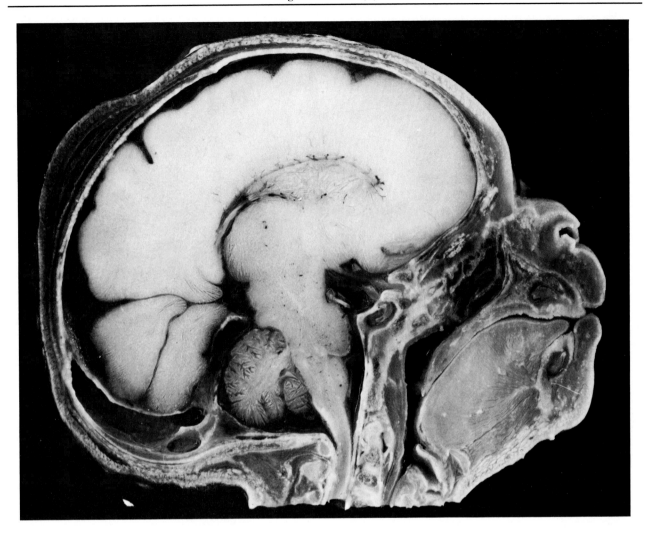

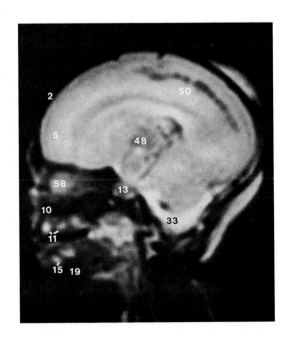

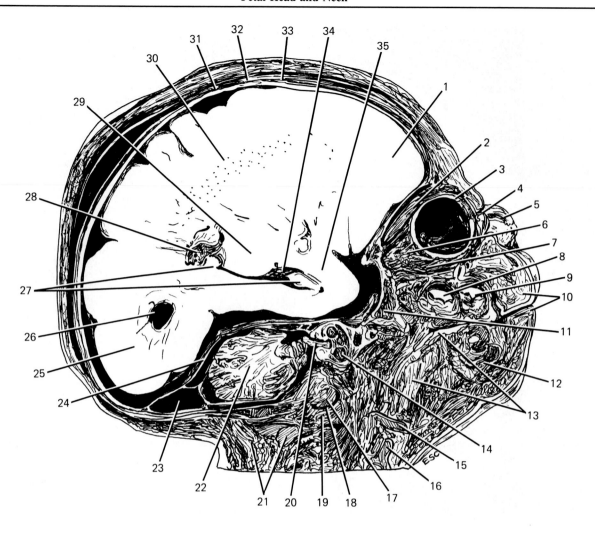

1–Frontal lobe
2–Superior rectus muscle
3–Sclera of right eyeball
4–Fused eyelids
5–Nose
6–Orbital fat
7–Inferior rectus muscle
8–2nd deciduous molar tooth
9–1st deciduous molar tooth
10–Lips
11–Sphenoid bone
12–Body of mandible
13–Tongue

14–Cochlea
15–Greater cornu of hyoid bone
16–Superior cornu of thyroid cartilage
17–Right occipital condyle
18–Atlanto-occipital joint
19–Lateral mass of atlas
20–Cochlear nerve entering modiolus of cochlea
21–Deep craniovertebral muscles
22–Right cerebellar hemisphere
23–Transverse sinus
24–Tentorium cerebelli
25–Occipital lobe

26–Posterior horn of lateral ventricle
27–Hippocampus
28–Choroid plexus in atrium of lateral ventricle
29–Thalamus
30–Parietal lobe
31–Parietal bone
32–Coronal suture
33–Frontal bone
34–Inferior horn of lateral ventricle
35–Temporal lobe
36–Atrium (trigone) of lateral ventricle
37–Vitreous of eyeball

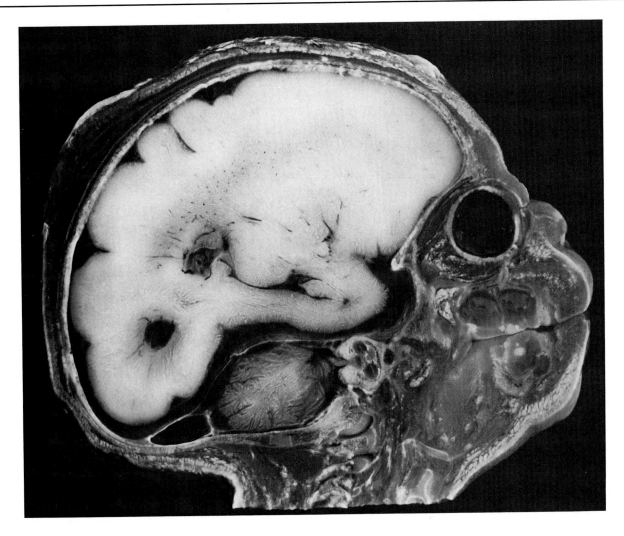

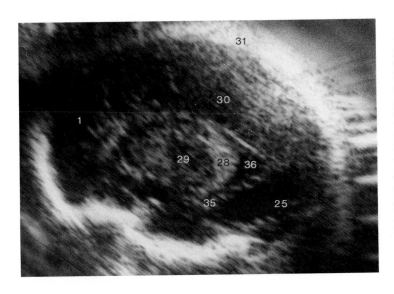

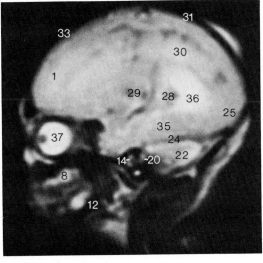

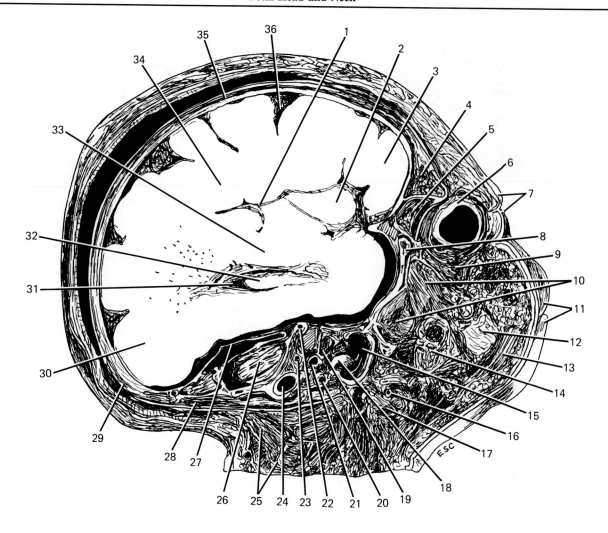

1–Lateral cerebral sulcus (Sylvian fissure)
2–Insula
3–Frontal lobe
4–Frontal bone
5–Lacrimal gland
6–Sclera of right eyeball
7–Fused eyelids
8–Greater wing of sphenoid bone
9–Orbital part of zygomatic bone
10–Temporalis muscle
11–Lips
12–Orbicularis oris muscle
13–Platysma muscle
14–Ramus of mandible

15–Tympanic cavity (middle ear)
16–External carotid artery
17–Stylohyoid muscle
18–Promontory (basal turn of cochlea)
19–Vestibule
20–Fenestra cochleae (round window)
21–Fenestra vestibuli (oval window)
22–Anterior semicircular canal
23–Lateral semicircular canal
24–Jugular bulb
25–Deep craniovertebral muscles
26–Cerebellum
27–Tentorium cerebelli
28–Lateral part of occipital bone
29–Squamous part of occipital bone

30–Occipital lobe
31–Inferior horn of lateral ventricle
32–Hippocampus
33–Temporal lobe
34–Parietal lobe
35–Parietal bone
36–Central sulcus (of Rolando)
37–Eyeball
38–Lens
39–Choroid plexus in atrium (trigone) of lateral ventricle
40–Crus commune
41–Superior semicircular canal
42–Petrous portion of temporal bone
43–Mouth

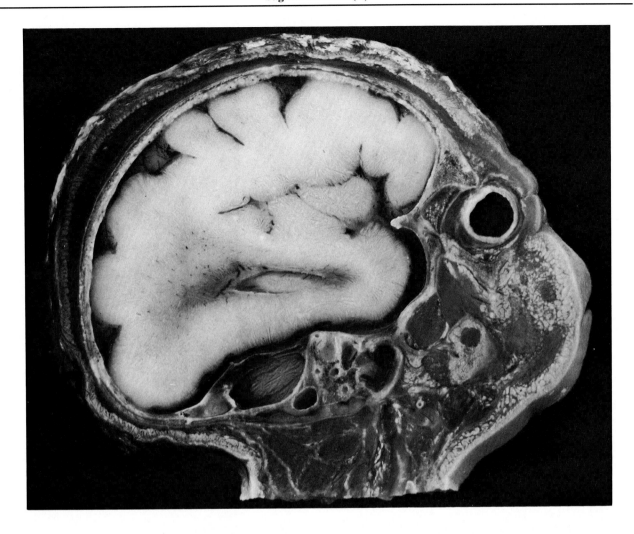

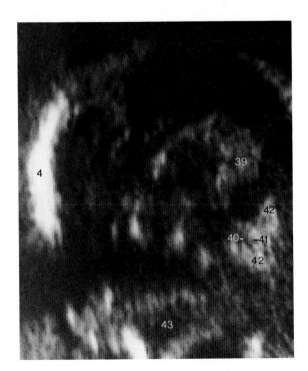

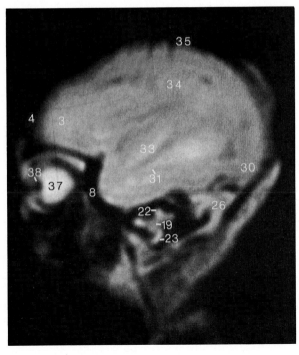

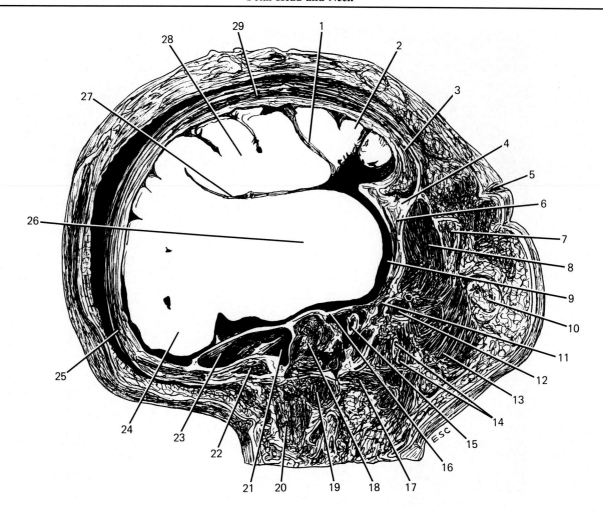

1–Central sulcus (of Rolando)
2–Frontal lobe
3–Frontal bone
4–Sphenoid fonticulus (fontanelle)
5–Lateral palpebral commissure
6–Squamous part of temporal bone
7–Zygomatic bone
8–Temporalis muscle
9–Middle cranial fossa
10–Buccal fat pad
11–Temporomandibular joint

12–Condylar process (head) of
      mandible
13–Masseter muscle
14–Maxillary artery and vein
15–Malleus and incus in tympanic
      cavity (middle ear)
16–Tegmen tympani
17–Stylohyoid muscles
18–Petrous part of temporal bone
19–Posterior belly of digastric muscle
20–Sternocleidomastoid muscle

21–Sigmoid sinus
22–Lateral part of occipital bone
23–Transverse sinus
24–Occipital lobe
25–Squamous part of occipital bone
26–Temporal lobe
27–Lateral cerebral sulcus (Sylvian
      fissure)
28–Parietal lobe
29–Parietal bone

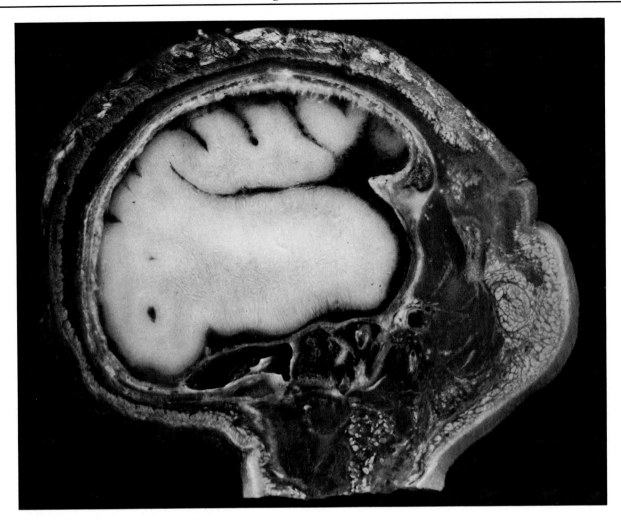

Fetal Head and Neck

SECTION 2

Coronal Sections

24 Week Fetus

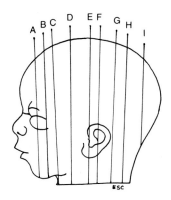

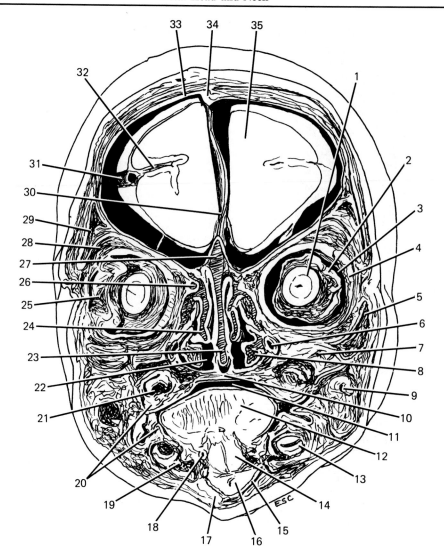

1–Lens of eyeball
2–Neural retina (detached)
3–Pigmented layer of retina
4–Sclera
5–Zygomatic bone
6–Left maxillary sinus
7–Maxilla
8–Inferior concha
9–Buccal fat pad
10–Hard palate
11–Oral cavity
12–Tongue
13–Lower deciduous canine tooth
14–Genioglossal muscle

15–Mylohyoid muscle
16–Geniohyoid muscle
17–Anterior belly of right digastric muscle
18–Submandibular duct
19–Mandible
20–Upper and lower gingivae
21–Upper deciduous canine tooth
22–Right nasal cavity
23–Nasal septum
24–Middle concha
25–Curve of sclera
26–Ethmoid cartilage
27–Crista galli

28–Orbit
29–Frontal bone
30–Falx cerebri
31–Superficial middle cerebral vein
32–Inferior frontal sulcus
33–Dura mater
34–Frontal suture
35–Frontal lobe
36–Closed eyelids
37–Vitreous of eyeball
38–Frontal bone
39–Periorbital fat

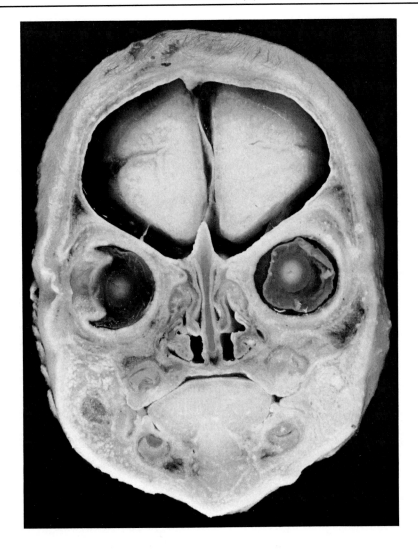

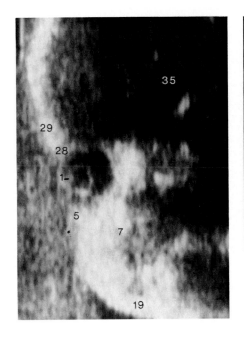
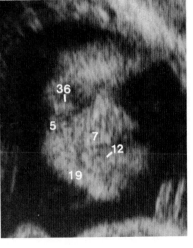
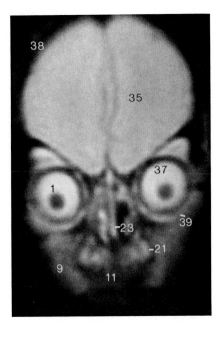

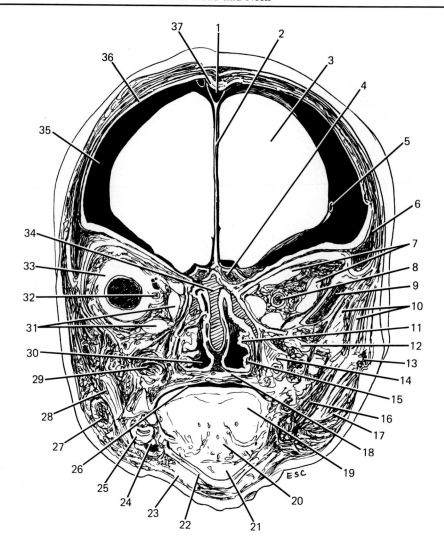

1–Superior sagittal sinus
2–Falx cerebri
3–Left frontal lobe
4–Olfactory bulb
5–Middle cerebral artery
6–Frontal bone
7–Extrinsic ocular muscles
8–Optic nerve
9–Zygomatic bone
10–Temporalis muscle
11–Middle concha
12–Fat in infratemporal fossa
13–Zygomatic bone (arch)
14–Maxilla
15–Inferior concha

16–Mandible
17–Masseter muscle
18–Hard palate
19–Tongue
20–Genioglossal muscle
21–Geniohyoid muscle
22–Mylohyoid muscle
23–Anterior belly of digastric muscle
24–Inferior alveolar nerve
25–Lower 2nd deciduous molar tooth
26–Oral cavity
27–Buccal fat pad
28–Masseter muscle
29–Upper 2nd deciduous molar tooth
30–Right nasal cavity

31–Ocular muscles
32–Optic nerve
33–Sclera
34–Nasal septum
35–Subdural space (artifactually
     enlarged)
36–Dura mater
37–Frontal suture
38–Lips
39–Lens of eyeball
40–Vitreous of eyeball
41–Periorbital fat
42–Cerebrospinal fluid

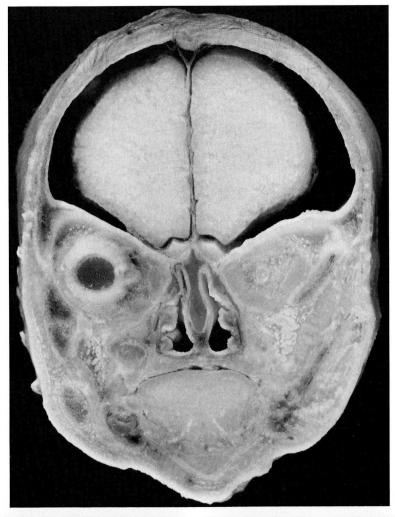

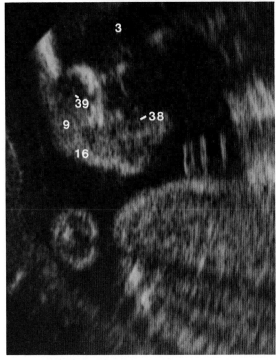

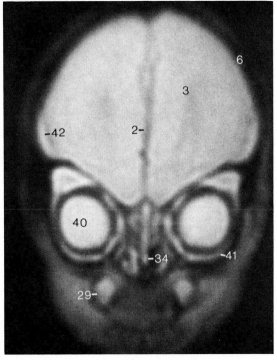

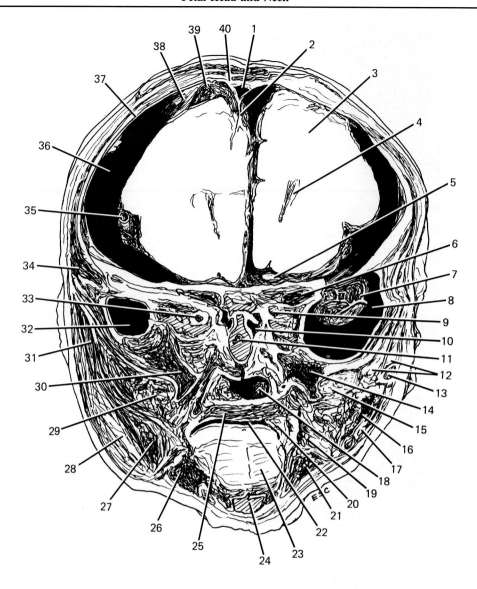

1–Superior sagittal sinus
2–Falx cerebri
3–Left frontal lobe
4–Anterior horn of lateral ventricle
   (collapsed)
5–Olfactory tract
6–Greater wing of sphenoid bone
7–Branch of middle cerebral artery
   on temporal lobe
8–Middle cranial fossa
9–Left optic nerve
10–Sphenoid concha
11–Body of sphenoid bone
12–Temporalis muscle
13–Zygomatic process of temporal
   bone

14–Base of pterygoid process of
   sphenoid bone
15–Lateral pterygoid muscle
16–Neck of mandible
17–Masseter muscle
18–Nasopharynx
19–Medial pterygoid muscle
20–Buccinator muscle
21–Left submandibular gland
22–Oral cavity
23–Tongue
24–Body of hyoid bone
25–Soft palate
26–Right submandibular gland
27–Body of mandible
28–Masseter muscle

29–Lateral pterygoid muscle
30–Greater wing of sphenoid bone
31–Temporalis muscle
32–Right middle cranial fossa
33–Optic nerve in posterior orbit
34–Frontal bone
35–Superficial middle cerebral vein
36–Subdural space (artifactually
   enlarged) of anterior cranial fossa
37–Dura mater
38–Arachnoid membrane
39–Subarachnoid space
40–Anterior fonticulus (fontanelle)
41–Cavum of septum pellucidum
42–Temporal lobe

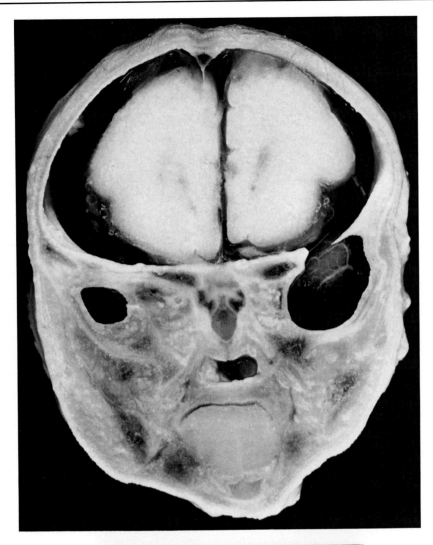

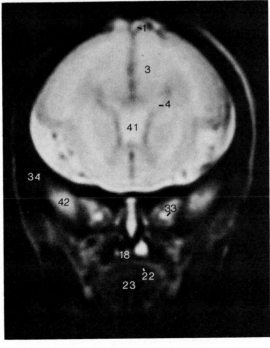

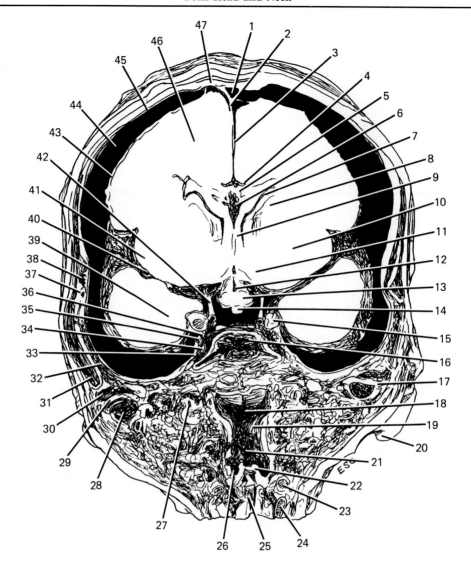

1–Superior sagittal sinus
2–Falx cerebri
3–Longitudinal cerebral fissure
4–Sulcus of corpus callosum
5–Corpus callosum
6–Cavum of septum pellucidum
7–Left lateral ventricle (collapsed)
8–Head of caudate nucleus
9–Stylus of septum pellucidum
10–Corpus striatum (basal nuclei or ganglia)
11–Olfactory area
12–3rd ventricle
13–Tuber cinereum
14–Infundibulum
15–Optic tract
16–Body of sphenoid bone
17–Articular disc of temporomandibular joint
18–Nasopharynx

19–Passavant fold or ridge
20–Left auricle
21–Oropharynx
22–Base of epiglottis
23–Greater cornu of hyoid bone
24–Superior cornu of thyroid cartilage
25–Interarytenoid notch
26–Right vallecula
27–Ascending palatine artery
28–Condylar process (head) of mandible
29–Articular disc of temporomandibular joint
30–Mandibular fossa of temporal bone
31–Temporalis muscle
32–Squamous part of temporal bone
33–Maxillary nerve (within lateral wall of cavernous sinus)
34–Abducens nerve (within cavernous sinus)

35–Ophthalmic nerve (within lateral wall of cavernous sinus)
36–Oculomotor and trochlear nerves (attached to lateral wall of cavernous sinus)
37–Sphenoid fonticulus (fontanelle)
38–Parietal bone
39–Amygdala of temporal lobe
40–Lateral cerebral fissure
41–Insula
42–Internal carotid artery
43–Arachnoid membrane (collapsed against pia mater which obliterates subarachnoid space)
44–Subdural space (artifactually enlarged)
45–Dura mater
46–Right parietal lobe
47–Anterior fonticulus (fontanelle)
48–Cerebrospinal fluid

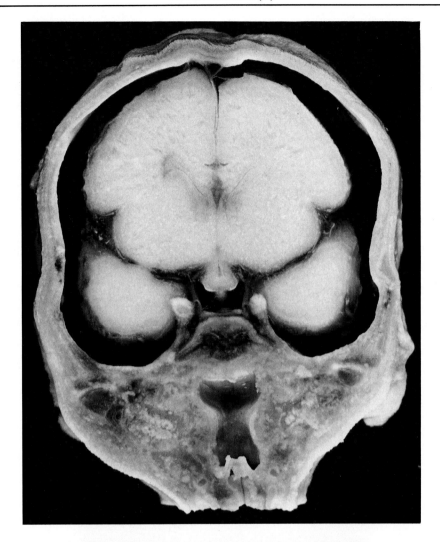

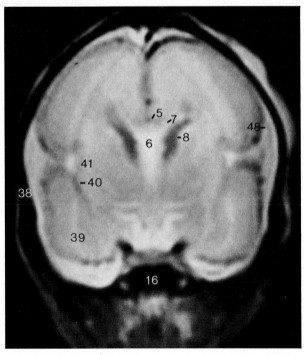

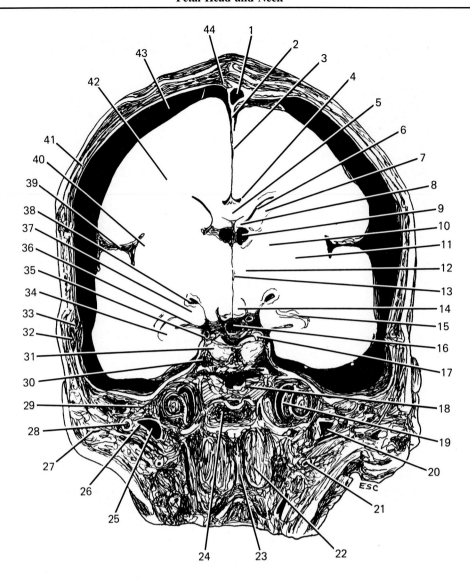

1–Superior sagittal sinus
2–Falx cerebri
3–Longitudinal cerebral fissure
4–Sulcus of corpus callosum
5–Corpus callosum
6–Lateral ventricle (collapsed)
7–Tail of caudate nucleus
8–Body of fornix
9–Left internal cerebral vein
10–Internal capsule
11–Corpus striatum (basal nuclei or ganglia)
12–Thalamus
13–3rd ventricle (collapsed)
14–Left mamillary body
15–Inferior horn of lateral ventricle
16–Interpeduncular cistern

17–Left oculomotor nerve
18–Cartilage of spheno-occipital synchondrosis
19–Left cochlea
20–Left tympanic cavity
21–Occipital artery
22–Left longus capitis muscle
23–Posterior wall of oropharynx
24–Basilar part of occipital bone
25–Right tympanic cavity
26–Tympanic membrane (ear drum)
27–External acoustic meatus
28–Malleus
29–Petrous part of temporal bone
30–Posterior extent of cavernous sinus
31–Right posterior clinoid process

32–Squamous part of temporal bone
33–Squamosal suture
34–Hippocampus
35–Posterior communicating artery of cerebral arterial circle
36–Hippocampal sulcus
37–Uncus
38–Choroid fissure
39–Lateral cerebral sulcus
40–Insula
41–Parietal bone
42–Right parietal lobe
43–Subdural space (artifactually enlarged)
44–Anterior fonticulus (fontanelle)
45–Cerebrospinal fluid

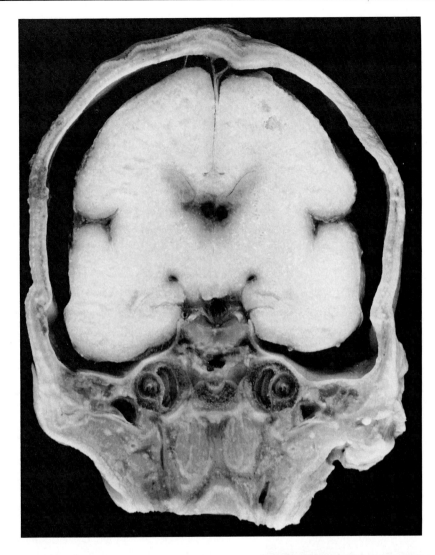

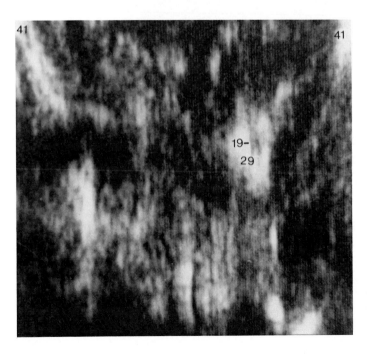

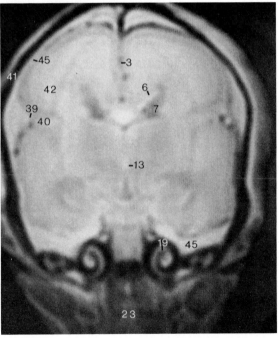

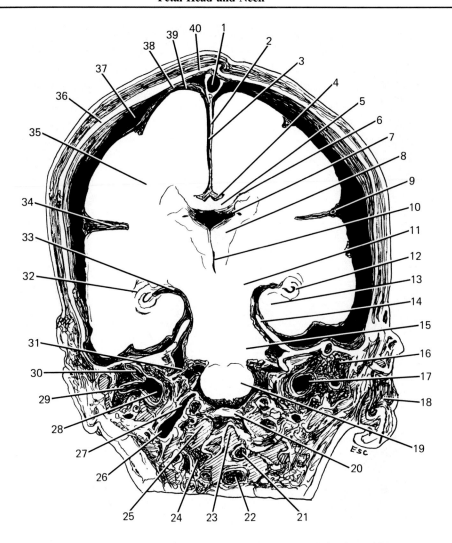

1–Superior sagittal sinus
2–Falx cerebri
3–Longitudinal cerebral fissure
4–Sulcus of corpus callosum
5–Corpus callosum
6–Left lateral ventricle (collapsed)
7–Internal cerebral veins joining to
 form great cerebral vein
8–Thalamus
9–Middle cerebral artery
10–3rd ventricle (collapsed)
11–Left cerebral peduncle
12–Hippocampus
13–Parahippocampal gyrus
14–Tentorium cerebelli
15–Middle cerebellar peduncle
16–Petrous portion of temporal bone

17–Left vestibule of inner ear
18–Auricle
19–Medulla oblongata
20–Anterior margin of foramen
 magnum
21–Ossification center of axis
22–Ossification center of C_3 vertebra
23–Dens of axis
24–Lateral mass of atlas
25–Right occipital condyle
26–Jugular fossa
27–Petro-occipital fissure
28–Right vestibule
29–Lateral semicircular canal
30–Anterior semicircular canal
31–Vestibulocochlear nerve entering
 internal acoustic meatus

32–Inferior horn of lateral ventricle
 (collapsed)
33–Choroid fissure
34–Lateral cerebral sulcus
35–Right parietal lobe
36–Dura mater
37–Subdural space (artifactually
 enlarged)
38–Arachnoid membrane
39–Subarachnoid space
40–Anterior fonticulus (fontanelle)
41–Parietal bone
42–Ear ridge—35 week gestation
43–Ear ridge—18 week gestation
44–Posterior semicircular canal

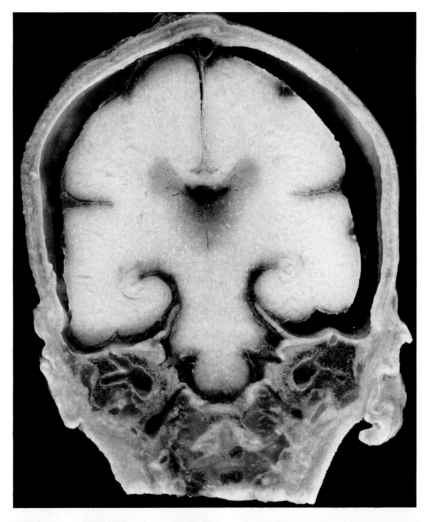

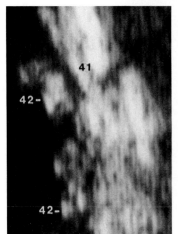

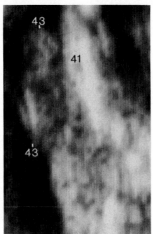

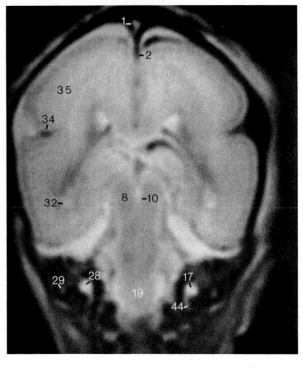

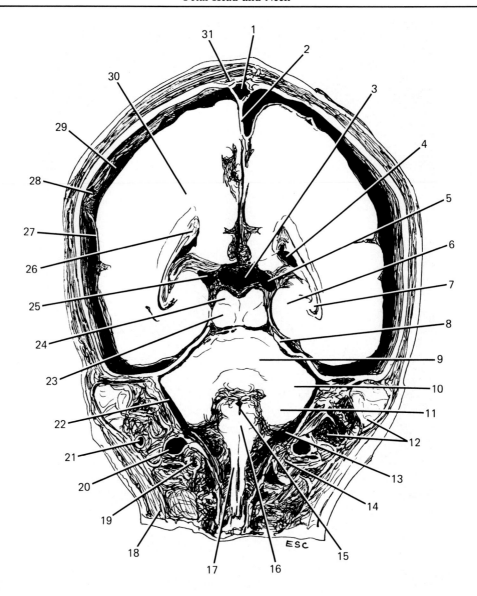

1–Superior sagittal sinus
2–Falx cerebri
3–Great cerebral vein
4–Left lateral ventricle
5–Left basilar vein
6–Thalamus
7–Hippocampus
8–Tentorium cerebelli
9–Superior cerebellar peduncle
10–Middle cerebellar peduncle
11–Left hemisphere of cerebellum
12–Temporal bone

13–Cerebellomedullaris cistern
14–Occipital bone
15–4th ventricle
16–Medulla oblongata
17–Spinal medulla (cord)
18–Sternocleidomastoid muscle
19–Posterior arch of atlas
20–Jugular bulb
21–Facial canal
22–Posterior cranial fossa
23–Inferior colliculus
24–Superior colliculus

25–Cistern of great cerebral vein
   (ambiens)
26–Choroid plexus of lateral ventricle
27–Arachnoid membrane in contact
   with pia mater (artifactually
   enlarges subdural space)
28–Arachnoid membrane in contact
   with dura mater as in life
29–Subarachnoid space
30–Right parietal lobe
31–Sagittal suture
32–Parietal bone

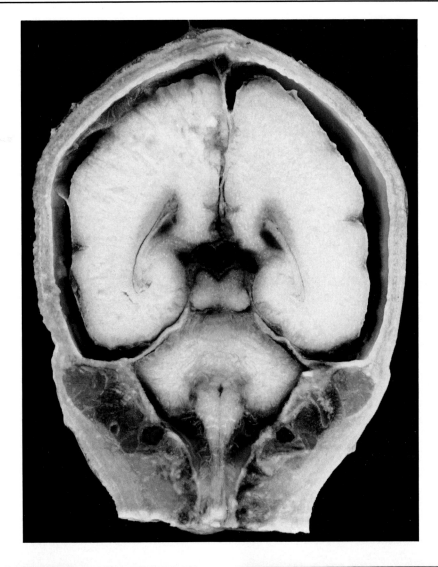

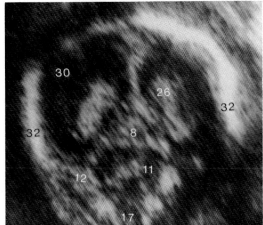

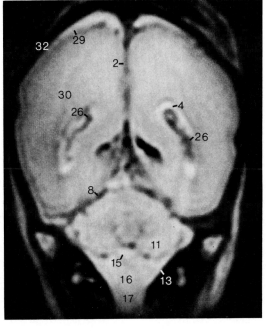

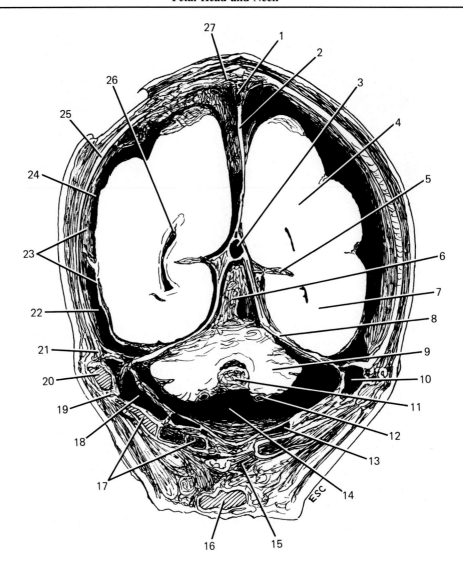

1–Superior sagittal sinus
2–Falx cerebri
3–Straight sinus
4–Left parietal lobe
5–Calcarine sulcus
6–Anterior vermis of cerebellum
7–Left occipital lobe
8–Tentorium cerebelli
9–Left hemisphere of cerebellum
10–Transverse sinus

11–Posterior vermis of cerebellum
12–Left posterior-inferior cerebellar
  artery
13–Posterior extent of jugular bulb
14–Cerebellomedullaris cistern
15–Posterior atlanto-occipital
  membrane
16–Posterior arch of atlas
17–Lateral part of occipital bone
18–Sigmoid sinus

19–Occipitomastoid suture
20–Temporal bone
21–Mastoid fonticulus (fontanelle)
22–Subdural space (artifactually
  enlarged)
23–Arachnoid membrane
24–Subarachnoid space
25–Right parietal bone
26–Inferior horn of lateral ventricle
27–Sagittal suture

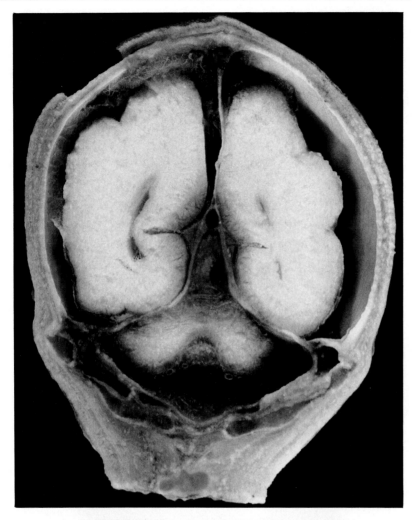

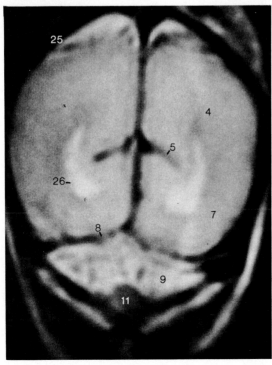

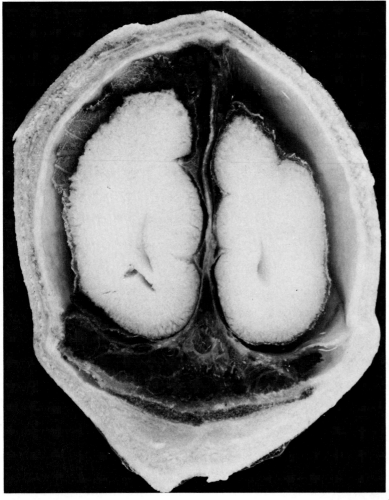

1–Superior or sagittal sinus
2–Falx cerebri
3–Left occipital lobe
4–Calcarine sulcus
5–Inferior horn of lateral ventricle
6–Tentorium cerebelli
7–Straight sinus
8–Left transverse sinus
9–Squamous part of occipital bone
10–Confluence of dural sinuses
11–Right semispinalis muscle
12–Right transverse sinus
13–Dura mater
14–Subdural space (artifactually enlarged)
15–Arachnoid membrane
16–Subarachnoid space
17–Sagittal suture

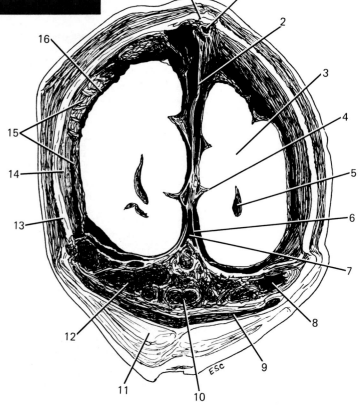

Fetal Head and Neck

SECTION 3

Axial Sections

30 Week Fetus

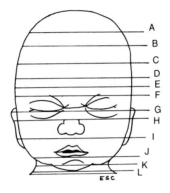

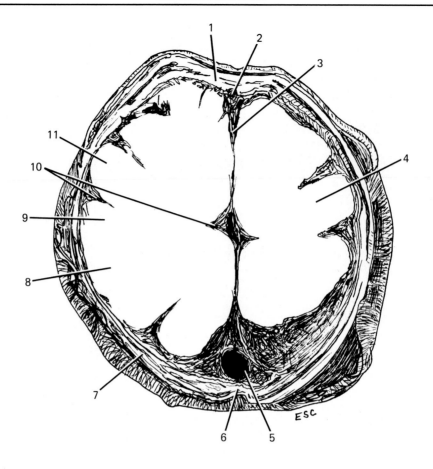

ESC

1–Anterior fonticulus (fontanelle)
2–Superior sagittal sinus
3–Falx cerebri
4–Left cerebral hemisphere

5–Superior sagittal sinus
6–Sagittal suture
7–Right parietal bone
8–Superior parietal lobule

9–Postcentral gyrus
10–Central sulcus (of Rolando)
11–Precentral gyrus

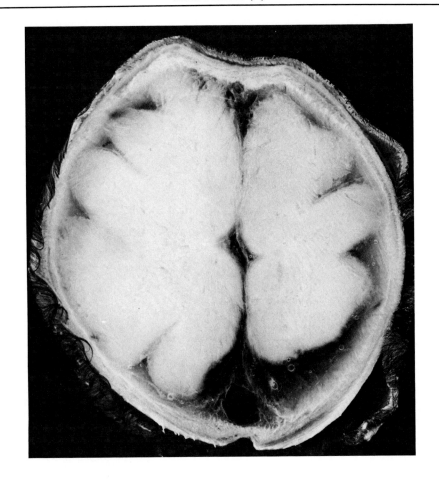

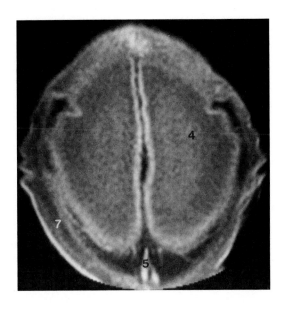

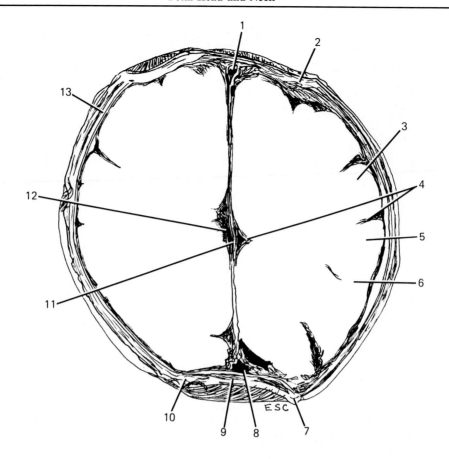

1–Superior sagittal sinus
2–Anterior fonticulus (fontanelle)
3–Precentral gyrus
4–Central sulcus (of Rolando)
5–Postcentral gyrus

6–Superior parietal lobule
7–Left lambdoidal suture
8–Superior sagittal sinus
9–Squamous part of occipital bone
10–Right lambdoidal suture

11–Falx cerebri
12–Longitudinal cerebral fissure
13–Right parietal bone
14–Falx/Interhemispheric fissure

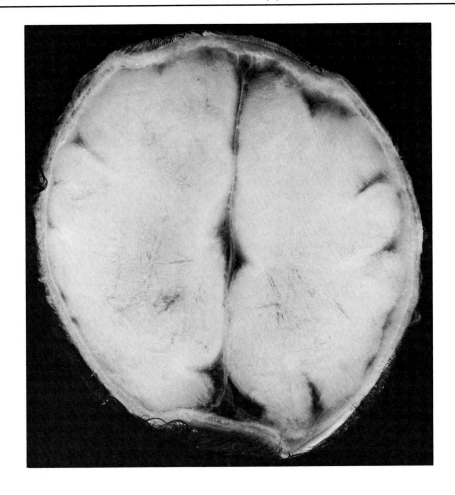

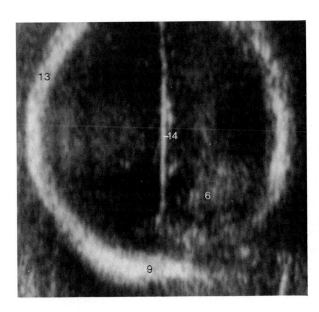

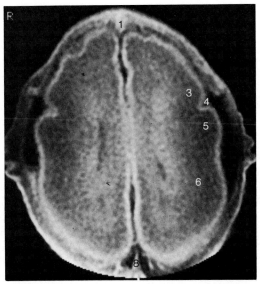

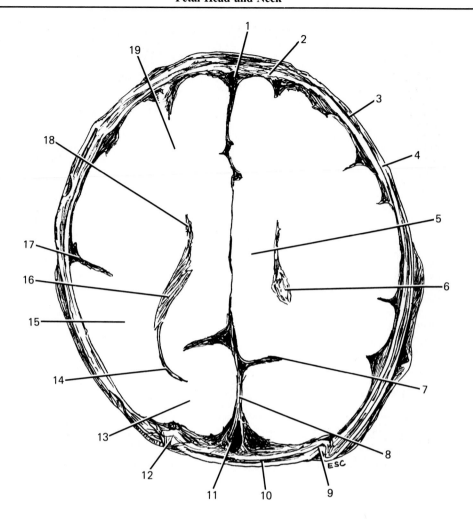

1–Superior sagittal sinus
2–Frontal (metopic) suture
3–Left frontal bone
4–Coronal suture
5–Cingulate gyrus
6–Central part of left lateral ventricle
7–Parieto-occipital sulcus
8–Falx cerebri

9–Left lambdoidal suture
10–Squamous part of occipital bone
11–Superior sagittal sinus
12–Right lambdoidal suture
13–Occipital lobe
14–Posterior (occipital) horn of lateral ventricle
15–Parietal lobe

16–Central part (body) of right lateral ventricle
17–Central sulcus (of Rolando)
18–Anterior (frontal) horn of lateral ventricle
19–Frontal lobe
20–Caudate nucleus

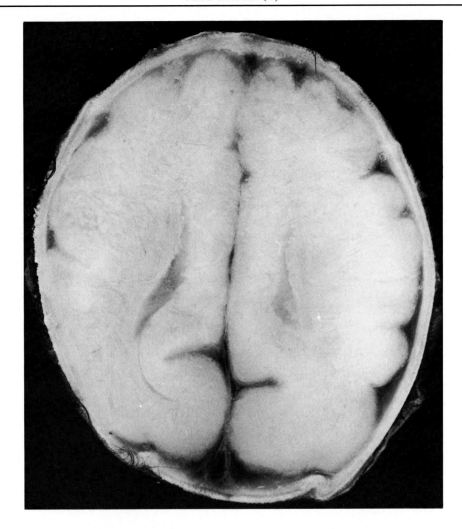

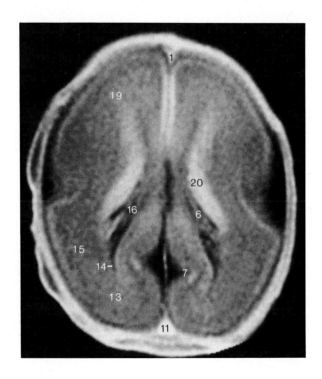

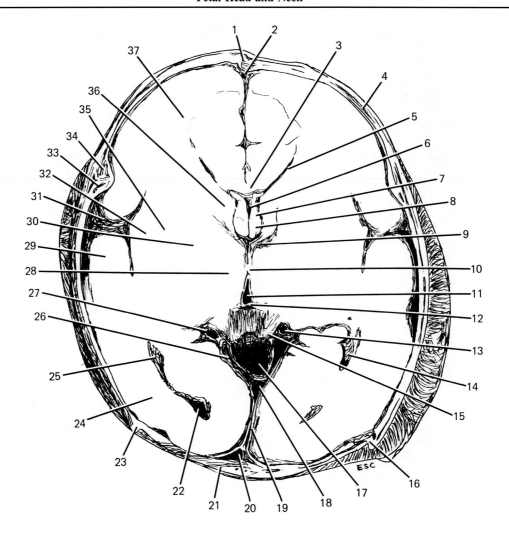

1–Frontal (metopic) suture
2–Superior sagittal sinus
3–Genu of corpus callosum
4–Left frontal bone
5–Anterior (frontal) horn of left lateral ventricle (collapsed)
6–Cavum of septum pellucidum
7–Stylus of septum pellucidum
8–Body of fornix
9–3rd ventricle
10–Interthalamic adhesion
11–3rd ventricle
12–Posterior commissure
13–Left internal cerebral vein
14–Choroid plexus in atrium of left lateral ventricle
15–Left superior colliculus

16–Left lambdoidal suture
17–Great cerebral vein
18–Straight sinus
19–Falx cerebri
20–Superior sagittal sinus
21–Lateral part of occipital bone
22–Posterior (occipital) horn of lateral ventricle
23–Right lambdoidal suture
24–Occipital lobe
25–Choroid plexus in atrium of right lateral ventricle
26–Cistern of great cerebral vein (ambiens)
27–Right internal cerebral vein
28–Thalamus
29–Temporal lobe

30–Internal capsule
31–Lateral cerebral sulcus (Sylvian fissure)
32–Insula
33–Parietal bone
34–Coronal suture
35–Corpus striatum (basal nuclei or ganglia)
36–Head of caudate nucleus
37–Frontal lobe
38–Lateral wall of frontal horn
39–Falx/Interhemispheric fissure
40–Hippocampus
41–Atrium (trigone) of lateral ventricle
42–Subarachnoid space

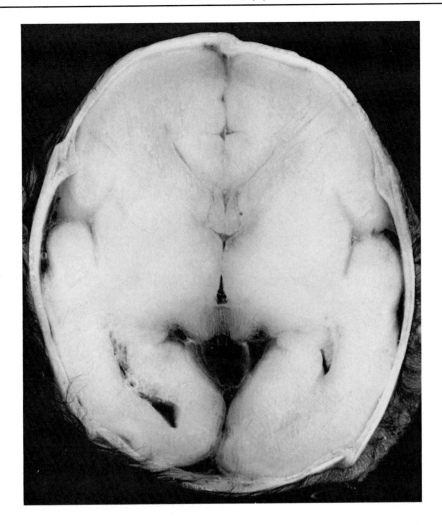

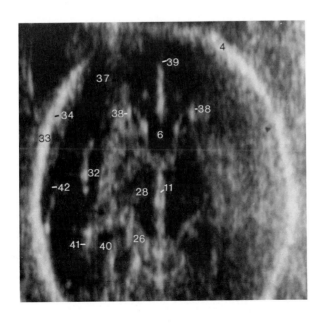

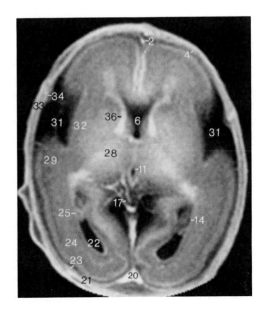

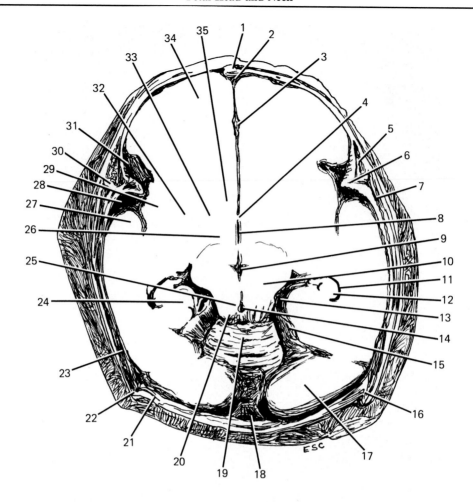

1–Frontal (metopic) suture
2–Superior sagittal sinus
3–Falx cerebri
4–Anterior commissure
5–Left frontal bone
6–Dura mater
7–Parietal bone
8–3rd ventricle
9–Interpeduncular fossa
10–Cerebral peduncle
11–Inferior (temporal) horn of lateral
    ventricle
12–Hippocampus
13–Choroid fissure
14–Cerebral aqueduct (of Sylvius)

15–Tentorium cerebelli
16–Lambdoidal suture
17–Occipital lobe
18–Confluence of sinuses
19–Cerebellum
20–Inferior colliculus
21–Squamous part of occipital bone
22–Lambdoidal suture
23–Parietal bone
24–Parahippocampal gyrus
25–Anulus (periaqueductal gray) of
    cerebral aqueduct
26–Thalamus
27–Temporal lobe
28–Middle cranial fossa

29–Insula
30–Coronal suture
31–Anterior cranial fossa
32–Corpus striatum (basal nuclei or
    ganglia)
33–Internal capsule
34–Frontal lobe
35–Head of caudate nucleus
36–Subarachnoid space
37–Posterior (occipital) horn of lateral
    ventricle
38–Great cerebral vein (of Galen)
39–Cistern of great cerebral vein
    (ambiens)

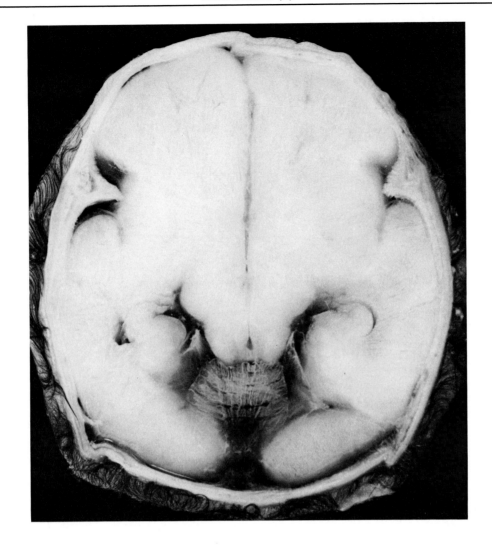

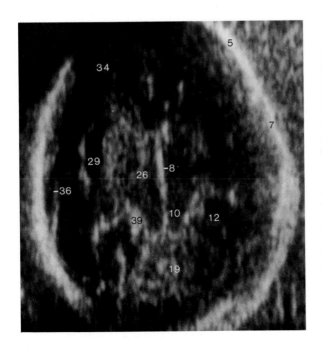

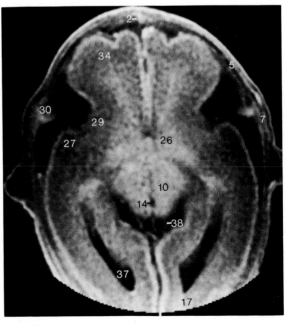

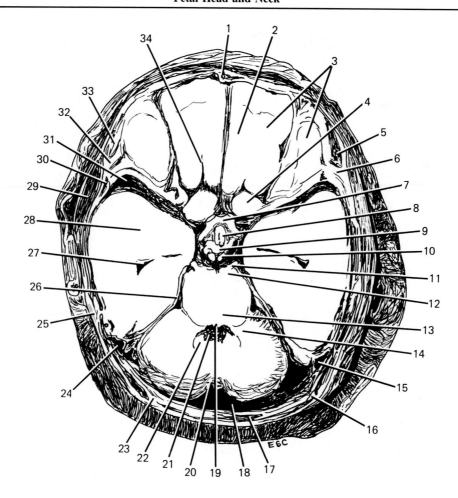

1–Frontal (metopic) suture
2–Straight (rectus) gyrus of left
   frontal lobe
3–Orbital gyri of frontal lobe
4–Anterior perforated substance
5–Frontal bone
6–Sphenoid fonticulus (fontanelle)
7–Optic chiasma
8–Infundibulum (pituitary stalk)
9–Tuber cinereum
10–Mamillary body
11–Oculomotor nerve
12–Pons
13–Medulla oblongata
14–Middle cerebellar peduncle
15–Transverse sinus

16–Lambdoidal suture
17–Squamous part of occipital bone
18–Cerebellomedullaris cistern
   (cisterna magna)
19–Median sulcus of medulla
   oblongata
20–Cerebellar pyramis
21–4th ventricle
22–Cerebellar tonsil
23–Lambdoidal suture
24–Transverse sinus
25–Mastoid fonticulus (fontanelle)
26–Tentorium cerebelli
27–Inferior (temporal) horn of lateral
   ventricle
28–Temporal lobe

29–Temporalis muscle
30–Parietal bone
31–Middle cranial fossa
32–Sphenoid fonticulus (fontanelle)
33–Frontal bone
34–Orbital sulcus
35–Anterior cerebral artery
36–Middle cerebral artery
37–Chiasmatic and interpeduncular
   cisterns (suprasellar cistern)
38–Basilar artery
39–Cerebellar hemisphere
40–Vermis of cerebellum
41–Midbrain/cerebral peduncle

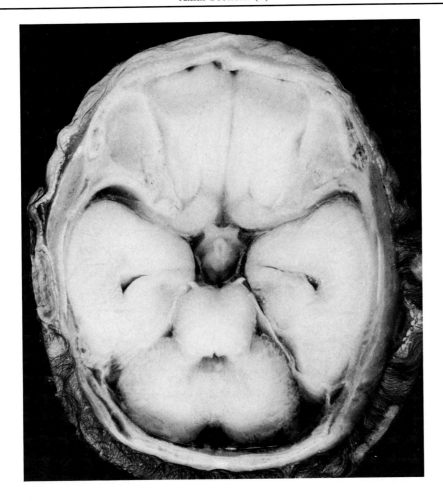

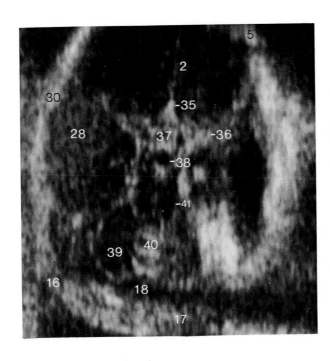

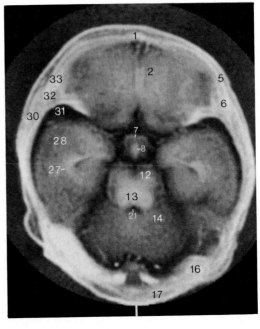

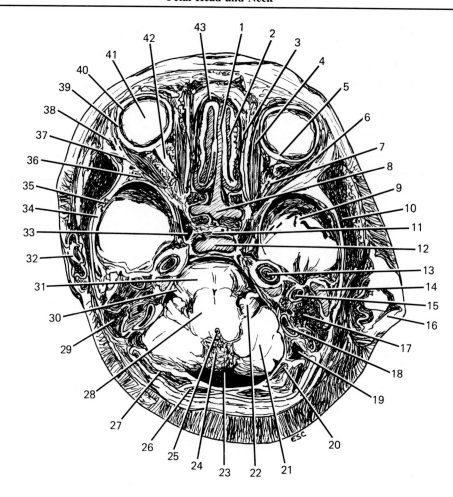

1–Nasal septum (cartilage)
2–Left nasal cavity
3–Ethmoid cartilage
4–Medial rectus muscle
5–Optic disc
6–Lateral rectus muscle
7–Orbital fat
8–Body of sphenoid bone (cartilage)
9–Middle cranial fossa
10–Temporalis muscle
11–Spheno-occipital synchondrosis
12–Basilar part of occipital bone
    (cartilage)
13–Cochlea
14–Left tympanic cavity (middle ear)
15–Vestibule
16–Left auricle
17–Petrous part of temporal bone

18–Posterior semicircular canal
19–Jugular bulb
20–Lateral part of occipital bone
21–Left cerebellar hemisphere
22–Flocculus
23–Cerebellomedullaris cistern
    (cisterna magna)
24–Uvula
25–4th ventricle
26–Trapezius muscle
27–Semispinalis capitis muscle
28–Medulla oblongata
29–Mastoid antrum
30–7th and 8th cranial nerves passing
    to internal acoustic meatus
31–Pons
32–Auricle
33–Cavernous sinus

34–Squamous part of temporal bone
35–Sphenosquamosal suture
36–Greater wing of sphenoid bone
37–Sphenozygomatic suture
38–Orbital part of zygomatic bone
39–Sclera
40–Pigmented layer of retina
41–Neural layer of retina
42–Optic nerve
43–Lateral nasal cartilage
44–Region of sella turcica
45–Anterior cranial fossa
46–Posterior cranial fossa
47–Lens
48–Vitreous of eyeball
49–Nasoethmoid complex
50–Orbit

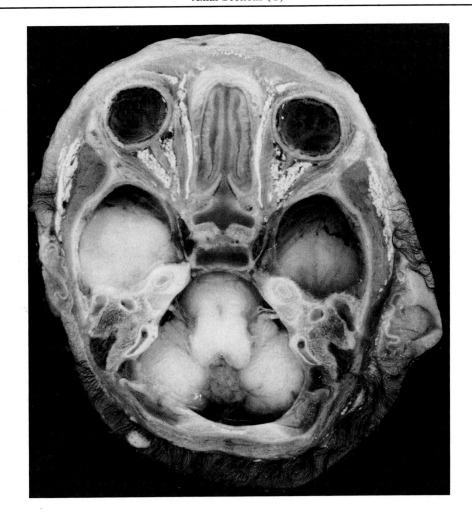

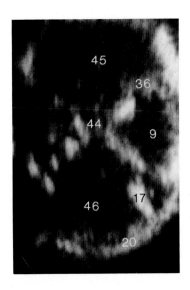

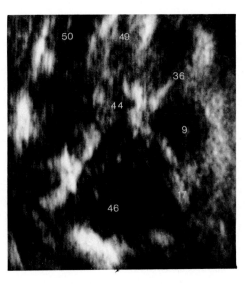

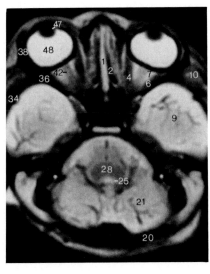

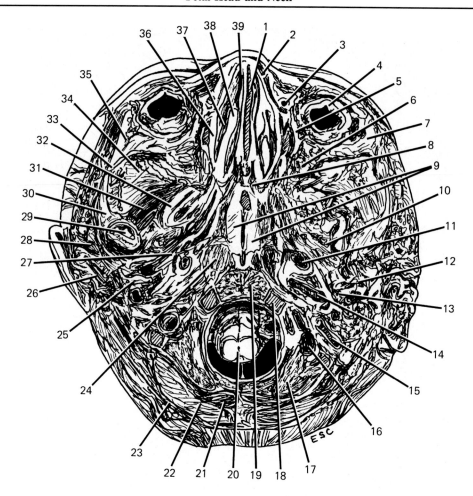

1–Nasal septum
2–Lateral nasal cartilage
3–Nasolacrimal duct
4–Left eyeball
5–Orbital part of maxilla
6–Inferior orbital fissure
7–Orbital part of zygomatic bone
8–Left choana
9–Roof of nasopharynx
10–Mandibular nerve
11–Internal carotid artery in carotid
canal
12–Malleus in tympanic cavity
(middle ear)
13–Stapedius muscle
14–Basal turn of cochlea
15–Posterior semicircular canal

16–Jugular fossa
17–Lateral part of occipital bone
18–Synchondrosis connecting basilar
and lateral parts of occipital bone
19–Basilar part of occipital bone
20–Medulla oblongata
21–Rectus capitis posterior major
muscle
22–Semispinalis capitis muscle
23–Trapezius muscle
24–Longus capitis muscle
25–External surface of tympanic
membrane (ear drum)
26–External acoustic meatus
27–Auditory (Eustachian) tube
28–Parotid gland

29–2nd deciduous molar tooth in
maxilla
30–Zygomatic process of temporal
bone
31–Lateral pterygoid muscle
32–Pterygoid process of sphenoid
bone
33–Temporozygomatic suture
34–Temporalis muscle
35–Orbital part of zygomatic bone
36–Ethmoid bone (cartilage)
37–Middle meatus
38–Middle concha
39–Right nasal cavity
40–Lens
41–Auricle of ear

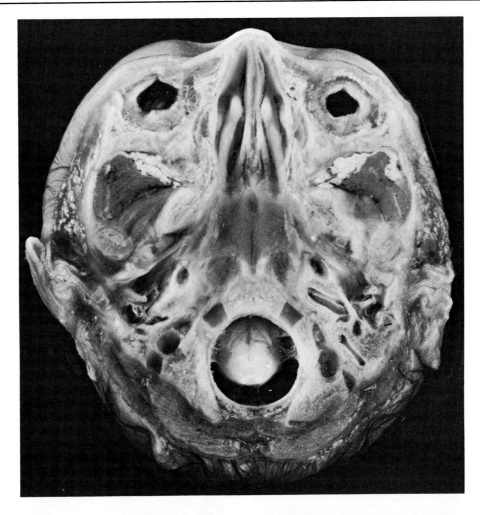

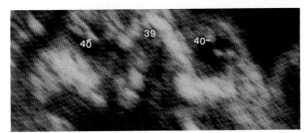

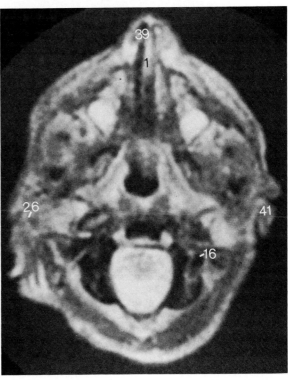

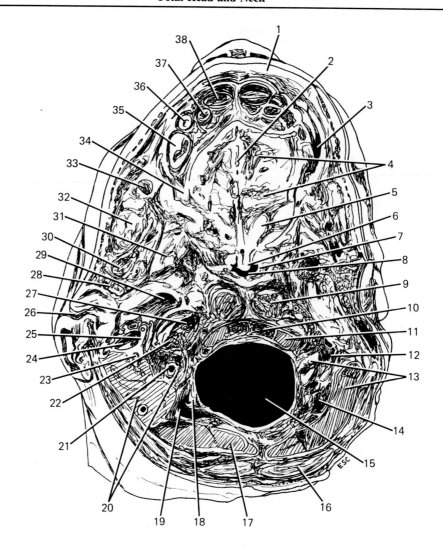

1–Superior labrum (upper lip)
2–Median raphe
3–Oral cavity
4–Hard palate
5–Soft palate
6–Uvula
7–Palatopharyngeal arch
8–Nasopharynx
9–Longus capitis muscle
10–Basilar part of occipital bone
11–Synchondrosis connecting basilar
    and lateral parts of occipital bone
12–Jugular bulb
13–Lateral part of occipital bone

14–Sigmoid sinus
15–Foramen magnum
16–Trapezius muscle
17–Lateral part of occipital bone
    (cartilage)
18–Dura mater
19–Sigmoid sinus
20–Temporal bone
21–Jugular bulb
22–Promontory of tympanic cavity
    (middle ear)
23–Facial nerve in facial canal
24–Tympanic membrane (ear drum)
25–Tympanic ring

26–Entrance of external acoustic
    meatus
27–Vestibule
28–Parotid gland
29–Auditory (Eustachian) tube
30–Neck of mandible
31–Medial pterygoid muscle
32–Masseter muscle
33–Coronoid process of mandible
34–Gingiva (gum)
35–1st deciduous upper molar tooth
36–Deciduous upper canine tooth
37–2nd deciduous upper incisor tooth
38–1st deciduous upper incisor tooth

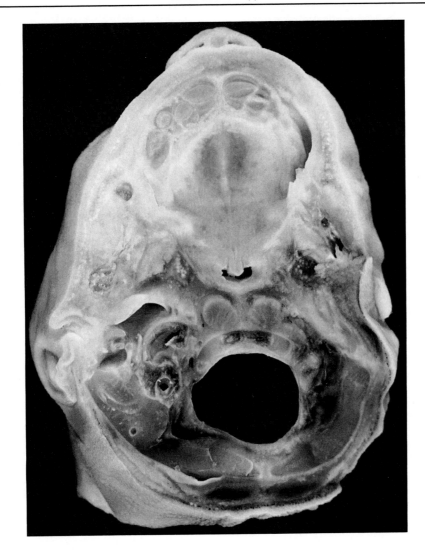

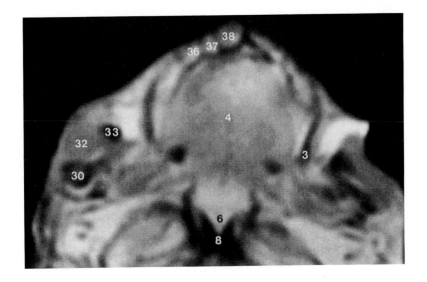

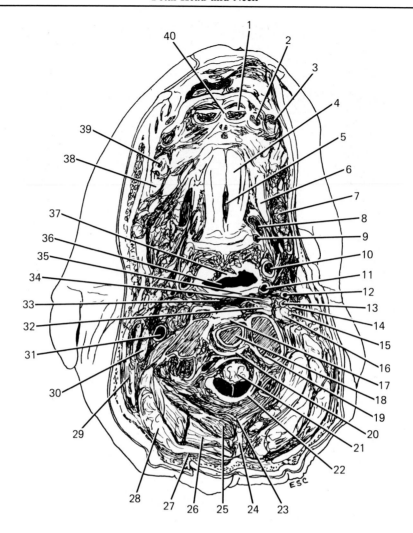

1–1st deciduous lower incisor tooth
2–2nd deciduous lower incisor tooth
3–Deciduous lower canine tooth
4–Geniohyoid muscle
5–Septum of tongue
6–Mylohyoid muscle
7–Submandibular gland
8–Hyoglossus muscle
9–Lesser cornu of hyoid bone
10–Greater cornu of hyoid bone
11–Superior cornu of thyroid cartilage
12–External carotid artery
13–Internal carotid artery
14–Vagus nerve

15–Internal jugular vein
16–Superior deep cervical lymph node
17–Anterior arch of atlas
18–Dens of axis
19–Lateral mass of atlas
20–Transverse ligament of atlas
21–Cervical spinal medulla (cord)
22–Dura mater
23–Tubercle of posterior arch of atlas
24–Ligamentum nuchae
25–Rectus capitis posterior minor
   muscle
26–Semispinalis capitis muscle
27–Trapezius muscle

28–Splenius capitis muscle
29–Sternocleidomastoid muscle
30–Posterior belly of digastric muscle
31–Right internal jugular vein
32–Longus capitis muscle
33–Retropharyngeal space
34–Superior sympathetic ganglion
35–Inferior pharyngeal constrictor
   muscle
36–Laryngopharynx
37–Epiglottis
38–2nd deciduous lower molar tooth
39–1st deciduous lower molar tooth
40–Symphysis of mandible

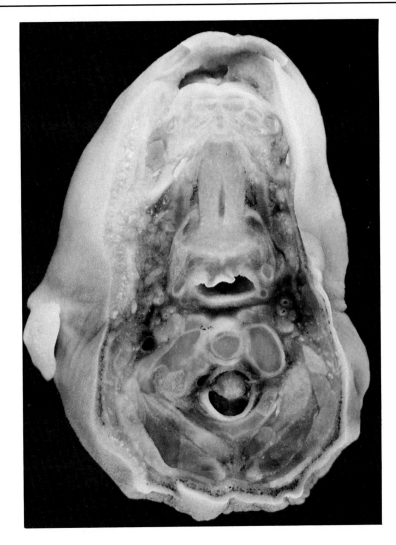

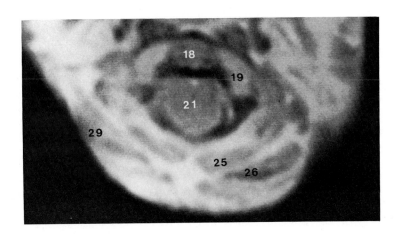

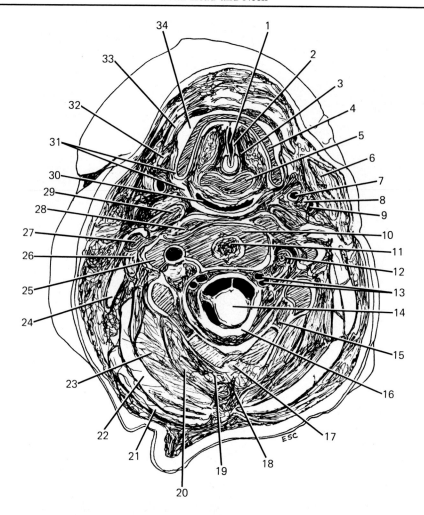

1–Rima glottidis (glottis)
2–Vocal fold (cord)
3–Vocalis part of thyroarytenoid muscle
4–Lamina of thyroid cartilage
5–Lamina of cricoid cartilage
6–Sternocleidomastoid muscle
7–Common carotid artery
8–Vagus nerve
9–Internal jugular vein
10–Body of 3rd cervical vertebra
11–Ossification center
12–Vertebral artery in transverse foramen

13–Anterior internal vertebral venous plexus
14–Cervical spinal medulla (cord)
15–Lamina of 3rd cervical vertebra
16–Dura mater
17–Spinous process
18–Ligamentum nuchae
19–Multifidi muscles
20–Semispinalis cervicis muscle
21–Trapezius
22–Splenius capitis muscle
23–Semispinalis capitis muscle
24–Levator scapulae muscle

25–Transverse process of 3rd cervical vertebra
26–Medial scalene muscle
27–Anterior scalene muscle
28–Longus colli muscle
29–Longus capitis muscle
30–Laryngopharynx
31–Inferior pharyngeal constrictor muscle
32–Omohyoid muscle
33–Sternohyoid muscle
34–Sternothyroid muscle

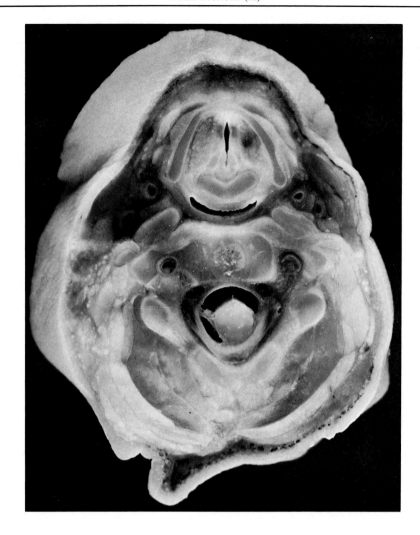

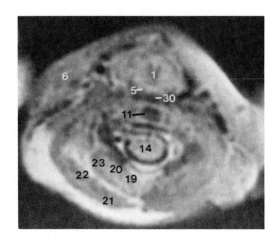

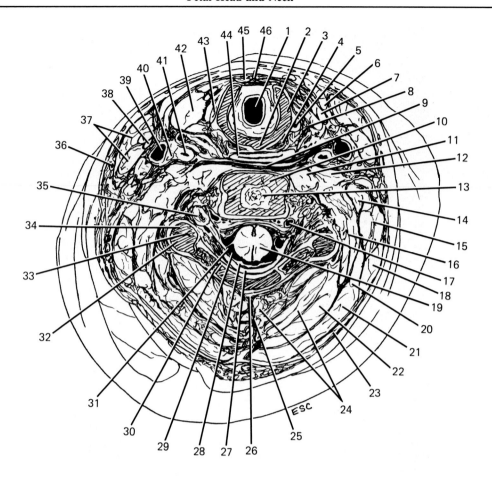

1–Infraglottic cavity of larynx
2–Lamina of cricoid cartilage
3–Arch of cricoid cartilage
4–Posterior cricoarytenoid muscle
5–Inferior cornu of thyroid cartilage
6–Sternohyoid muscle
7–Sternothyroid muscle
8–Left lateral lobe of thyroid gland
9–Prevertebral fascial cleft
10–Body of 4th cervical vertebra
11–Longus colli muscle
12–Longus capitis muscle
13–Ossification center
14–Anterior scalene muscle
15–Middle scalene muscle
16–Posterior scalene muscle
17–Anterior interior vertebral venous
    plexus

18–Levator scapulae muscle
19–Cervical spinal medulla (cord)
20–Splenius cervicis muscle
21–Splenius capitis muscle
22–Semispinalis capitis muscle
23–Trapezius muscle
24–Spinalis cervicis and multifidi
    muscles
25–Ligamentum nuchae
26–Spinous process of 4th cervical
    vertebra
27–Dura mater
28–Arachnoid membrane
29–Subarachnoid space
30–Lamina of 4th cervical vertebra
31–Denticulate ligament
32–Inferior articular process of 4th
    cervical vertebra

33–Articular cavity
34–Superior articular process of 5th
    cervical vertebra
35–Dorsal spinal ganglion of 5th
    cervical spinal nerve (in
    intervertebral foramen)
36–External jugular vein
37–Sternocleidomastoid muscle
38–Intermediate tendon of mylohyoid
    muscle
39–Internal jugular vein
40–Vagus nerve
41–Common carotid artery
42–Right lateral lobe of thyroid gland
43–Cricothyroid muscle
44–Esophagus
45–Isthmus of thyroid gland
46–Inferior thyroid vein

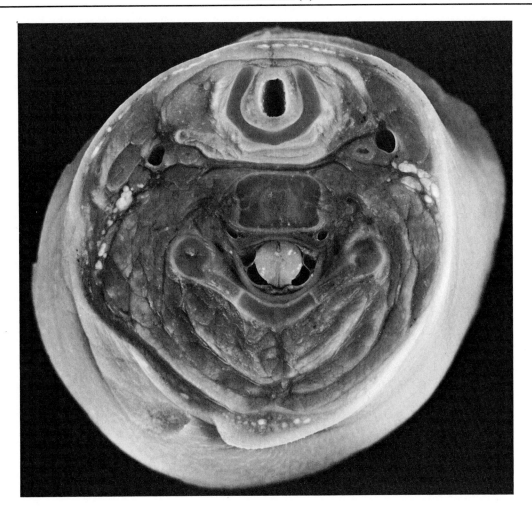

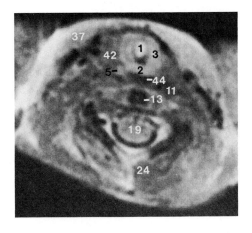

Fetal Thorax and Abdomen

SECTION 1

Axial Sections

20 Week Fetus

Male Thorax and Abdomen

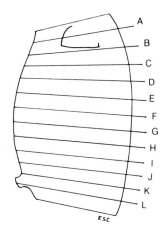

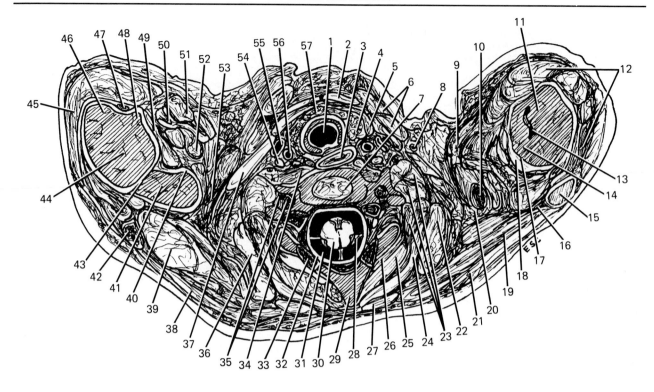

1–Trachea
2–Sternohyoid muscle
3–Esophagus
4–Left lateral lobe of thyroid gland
5–Sternothyroid muscle
6–Sternocleidomastoid muscle
7–Body of 6th cervical vertebra
8–External jugular vein
9–Pectoralis major muscle
10–Clavicle
11–Greater tubercle of humerus
12–Deltoid muscle
13–Anatomical neck of humerus
14–Head of humerus
15–Acromion
16–Spine of scapula
17–Glenoid cavity
18–Glenoid labrum
19–Supraspinatus muscle
20–Subclavius muscle
21–Trapezius muscle
22–Levator scapulae muscle
23–Anterior, middle and posterior
scalene muscles

24–Splenius capitis muscle
25–Semispinalis capitis muscle
26–Semispinalis cervicis and multifidi
muscles
27–Serratus posterior superior muscle
28–Denticulate ligament
29–Spinous process
30–Spinal medulla (cord)
31–Subarachnoid space
32–Dura mater
33–Ossification center of lamina of
6th cervical vertebra
34–Longus colli muscle
35–Vertebral vein and artery in
transverse foramen of transverse
process
36–Levator scapulae muscle
37–Inferior belly of omohyoid muscle
38–Trapezius muscle
39–Infraspinatus muscle
40–Coracoid process
41–Neck of scapula
42–Spine of scapula
43–Glenoid cavity

44–Head of humerus
45–Deltoid muscle
46–Greater tubercle of humerus
47–Long head of biceps brachii
muscle in intertubercular groove
48–Lesser tubercle
49–Subscapularis muscle
50–Coracobrachialis muscle
51–Pectoralis major muscle
52–Pectoralis minor muscle
53–Clavicle
54–Vagus nerve
55–Internal jugular vein
56–Common carotid artery
57–Isthmus of thyroid gland
58–Body of 1st thoracic vertebra
59–Lamina of 1st thoracic vertebra
60–Proximal end of 1st rib
61–Superior lobe of left lung
62–Cerebrospinal fluid

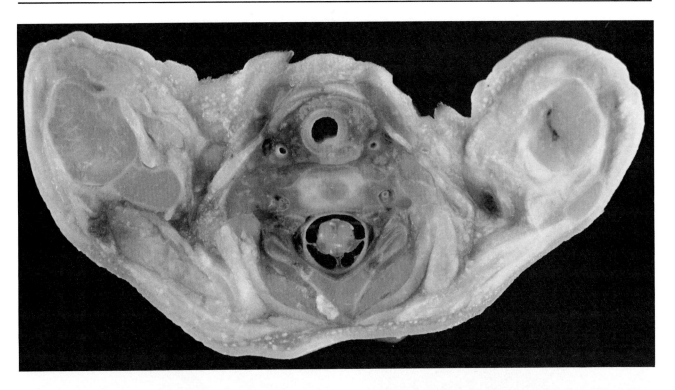

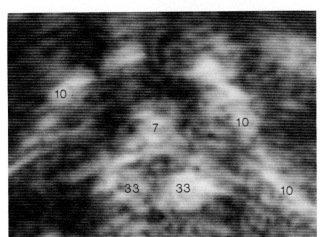

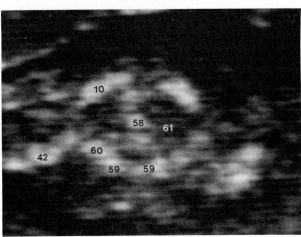

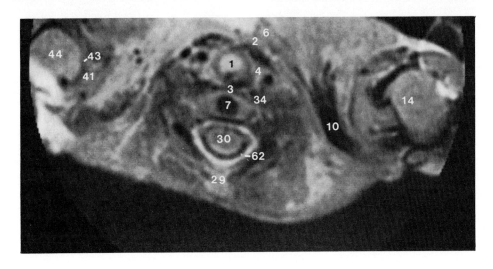

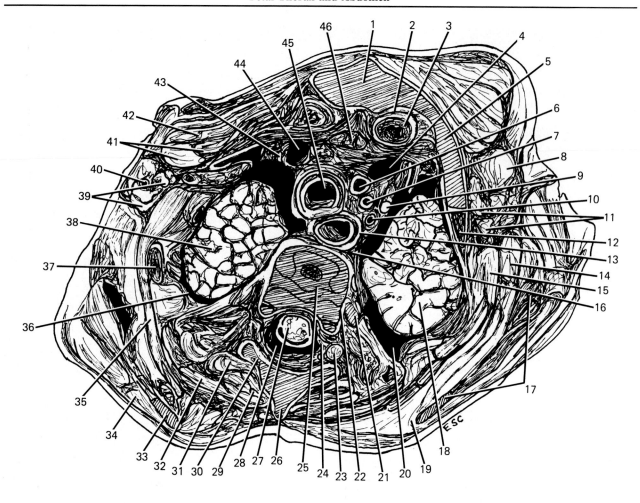

1–Manubrium of sternum
2–Sternoclavicular joint
3–Left clavicle
4–Left brachiocephalic vein
5–1st costal cartilage
6–Brachiocephalic artery
7–Left common carotid artery
8–Pectoralis minor muscle
9–Left vagus nerve
10–Left subclavian artery
11–Brachial plexus nerves
12–Left 1st rib
13–Esophagus
14–Subscapularis muscle
15–Serratus anterior muscle
16–Thoracic duct
17–Left scapula

18–Superior lobe of left lung
19–Trapezius muscle
20–Left pleural cavity
21–Head of 2nd rib
22–Costovertebral joint
23–Dorsal spinal ganglion in
    intervertebral foramen
24–Roots of T_2 spinal nerve
25–Body of T_2 vertebra
26–Spinous process of T_2 vertebra
27–Spinal medulla (cord)
28–Subarachnoid space
29–Semispinalis capitis muscle
30–Lamina of T_2 vertebra
31–Semispinalis cervicis and multifidi
    muscles
32–Splenius capitis muscle

33–Right scapula
34–Infraspinatus muscle
35–Right serratus anterior muscle
36–Right pleural cavity
37–Right 2nd rib
38–Superior lobe of right lung
39–Brachial plexus nerves
40–Axillary artery
41–Right pectoralis minor muscle
42–Right pectoralis major muscle
43–Right vagus nerve
44–Right brachiocephalic vein
45–Trachea
46–Thymus gland

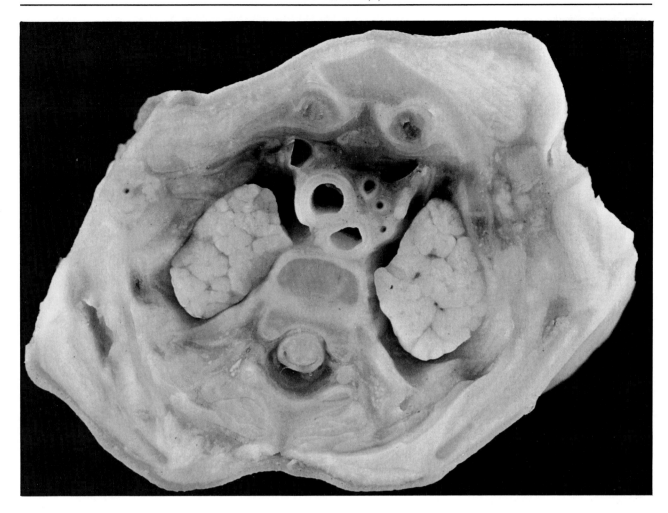

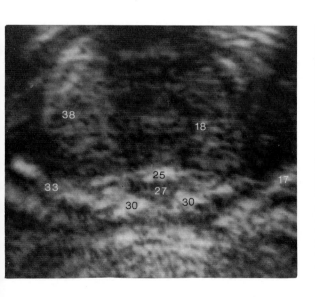

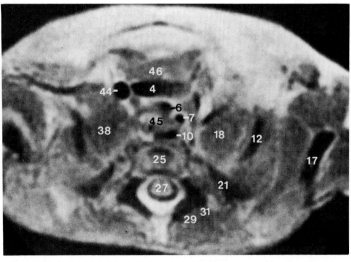

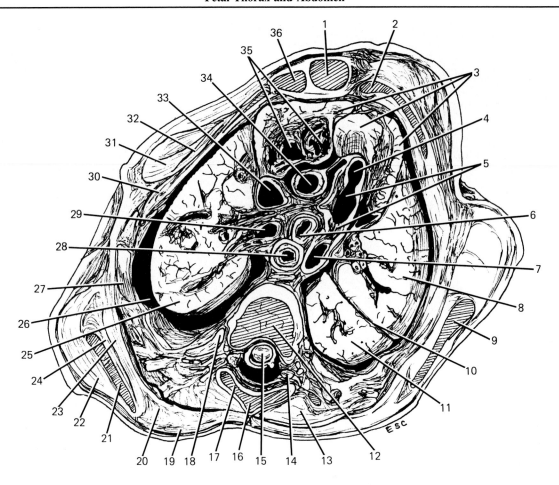

1–Body of sternum
2–Left 2nd costal cartilage
3–Thymus gland
4–Pulmonary trunk
5–Ductus arteriosus
6–Left main bronchus
7–Descending aorta
8–Superior lobe of left lung
9–Left scapula
10–Oblique fissure
11–Inferior lobe of left lung
12–Body of T$_4$ vertebra
13–Semispinalis thoracis, multifidi, longissimus thoracis and iliocostalis thoracis muscles

14–Dorsal ganglion of T$_4$ spinal nerve
15–Spinal medulla (cord)
16–Spinous process of T$_4$ vertebra
17–Lamina of T$_4$ vertebra
18–Head of 4th rib
19–Trapezius muscle
20–Rhomboideus major muscle
21–Right scapula
22–Teres major muscle
23–Serratus anterior muscle
24–Subscapularis muscle
25–Superior lobe of right lung
26–Pleural cavity (artifactually enlarged)

27–3rd rib
28–Esophagus
29–Right main bronchus
30–Intercostal muscles
31–Pectoralis major muscle
32–Pectoralis minor muscle
33–Superior vena cava
34–Ascending aorta
35–Left brachiocephalic vein
36–Right 2nd costal cartilage

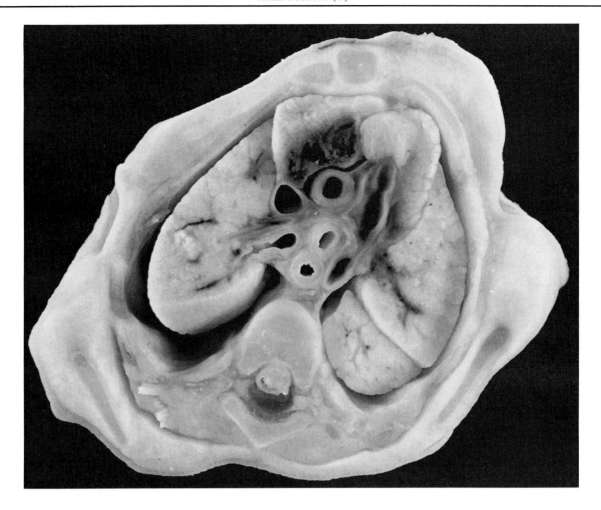

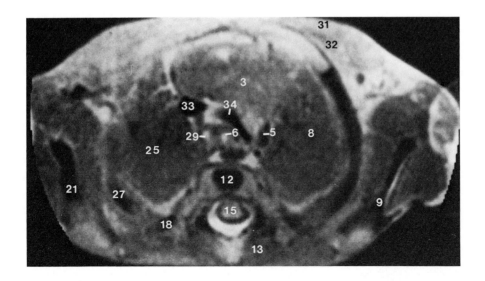

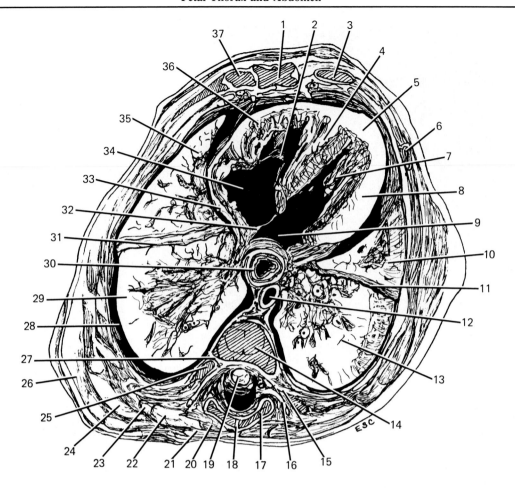

1–Body of sternum
2–Cusp of right atrioventricular
   valve
3–Left 4th costal cartilage
4–Interventricular septum
5–Apex of heart
6–4th rib
7–Papillary muscle
8–Left ventricle
9–Left atrium
10–Superior lobe of left lung
11–Oblique fissure
12–Descending thoracic aorta
13–Inferior lobe of left lung

14–Body of T$_8$ vertebra
15–8th intercostal nerve
16–Dorsal ramus of T$_8$ spinal nerve
17–Lamina of T$_8$ vertebra
18–Spinous process of T$_8$ vertebra
19–Spinal medulla (cord)
20–Semispinalis thoracis and multifidi
    muscles
21–Trapezius muscle
22–Longissimus thoracis muscle
23–Iliocostalis thoracis muscle
24–Serratus anterior muscle
25–Head of 8th rib
26–Latissimus dorsi muscle

27–Costovertebral joint
28–Right pleural cavity (artifactually
    enlarged)
29–Inferior lobe of right lung
30–Esophagus
31–Oblique fissure
32–Interatrial septum
33–Right phrenic nerve
34–Right atrium
35–Middle lobe of right lung
36–Right ventricle
37–Right 5th costal cartilage
38–Left atrioventricular valve

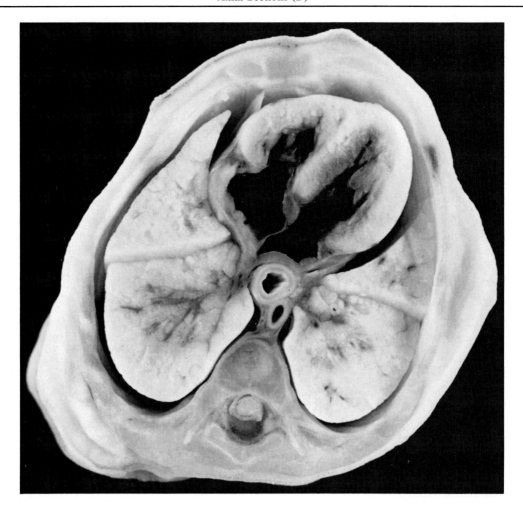

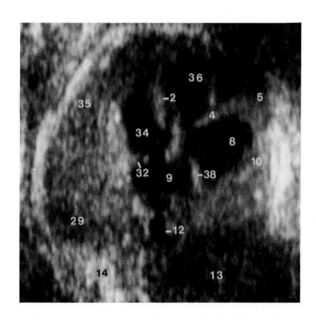

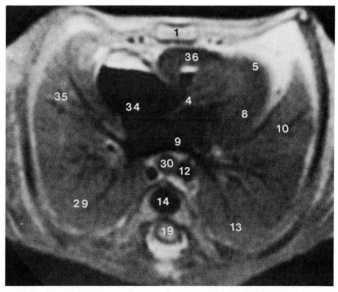

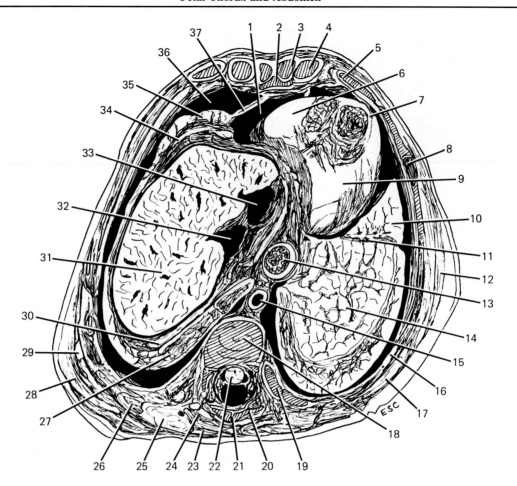

1–Pericardial cavity
2–Xiphoid process of sternum
3–Left 7th costal cartilage
4–6th costal cartilage
5–5th costal cartilage
6–Right ventricle
7–Apex of heart
8–5th rib
9–Left ventricle
10–Superior lobe of left lung
11–Oblique fissure
12–Left latissimus dorsi muscle
13–Esophagus
14–Inferior lobe of left lung

15–Descending thoracic aorta
16–Intercostal muscles
17–Serratus anterior muscle
18–Body of T_9 vertebra
19–Head of 9th rib
20–Lamina of T_9 vertebra
21–Spinous process of T_9 vertebra
22–Spinal medulla (cord)
23–Trapezius muscle
24–Semispinalis thoracis and multifidi muscles
25–Longissimus thoracis muscle
26–Iliocostalis thoracis muscle
27–Inferior lobe of right lung

28–Latissimus dorsi muscle
29–Serratus anterior muscle
30–Diaphragm
31–Right lobe of liver
32–Inferior vena cava
33–Ductus venosus
34–Diaphragm
35–Middle lobe of right lung
36–Right pleural cavity (artifactually enlarged)
37–Fused mediastinal pleura and pericardium
38–Left lobe of liver

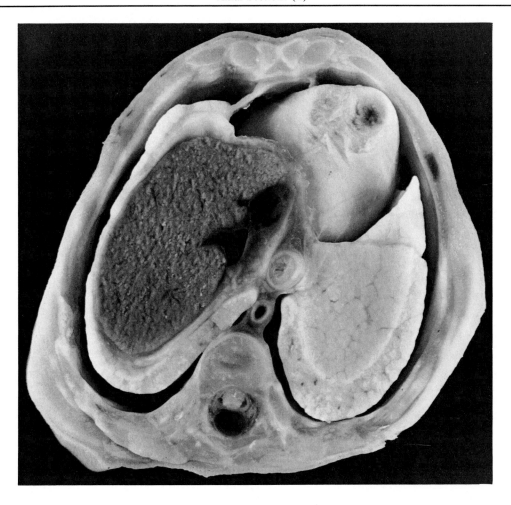

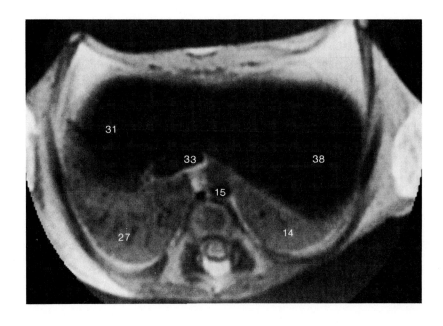

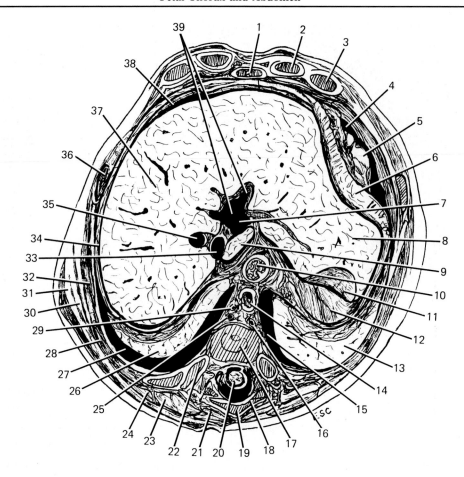

1–Xiphoid process of sternum
2–7th costal cartilage
3–6th costal cartilage
4–Pericardial cavity
5–Apex of heart
6–Diaphragm
7–Opening of left hepatic vein
8–Left lobe of liver
9–Caudate lobe of the liver
10–Esophagus
11–Gastric (fundic) impression of liver
12–Gastric (fundic) impression of diaphragm
13–Inferior lobe of left lung
14–Descending thoracic aorta

15–Left pleural cavity (artifactually enlarged)
16–Hemiazygous vein
17–Body of T_{10} vertebra
18–Lamina of T_{10} vertebra
19–Spinous process of T_{10} vertebra
20–Spinal medulla
21–Semispinalis thoracis and multifidi muscles
22–Head of the 10th rib
23–Longissimus thoracis muscle
24–Iliocostalis lumborum muscle
25–Azygous vein
26–Inferior lobe of right lung

27–Right pleural cavity (artifactually enlarged)
28–9th rib
29–Thoracic duct
30–Serratus anterior muscle
31–Latissimus dorsi muscle
32–8th rib
33–Inferior vena cava
34–Diaphragm
35–Right hepatic vein
36–7th rib
37–Right lobe of liver
38–Peritoneal cavity
39–Ductus venosus

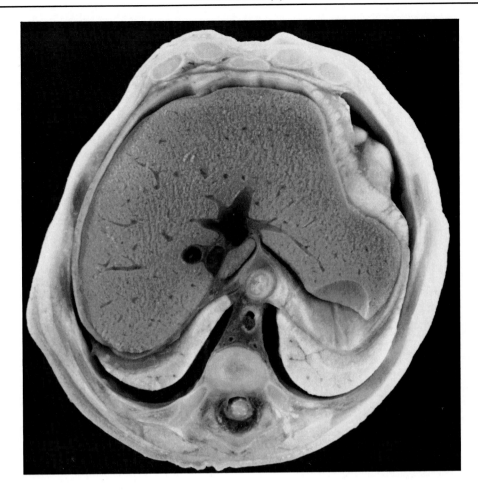

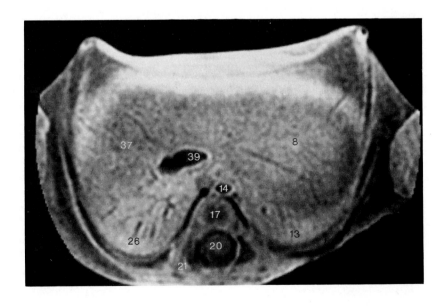

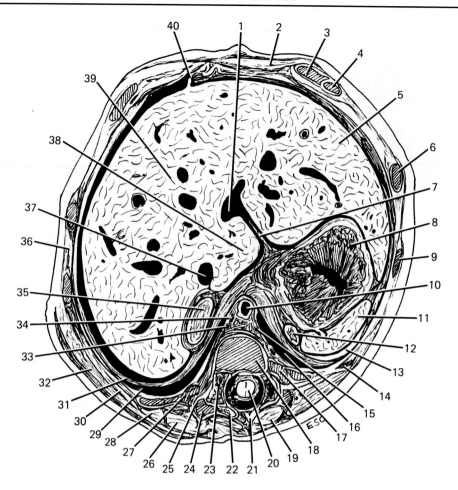

1–Left branch of portal vein
2–Left rectus abdominis muscle
3–8th costal cartilage
4–7th costal cartilage
5–Left lobe of liver
6–8th rib
7–Lesser omentum
8–Stomach
9–9th rib
10–Descending thoracic aorta
11–Spleen
12–Left suprarenal gland
13–Diaphragm
14–10th rib
15–Hemiazygous vein

16–Left costodiaphragmatic pleural recess (artifactually enlarged)
17–Head of 11th rib
18–Body of T_{11} vertebra
19–Semispinalis thoracis and multifidi muscles
20–Spinal medulla (cord)
21–Spinous process of T_{11} vertebra
22–Lamina of T_{11} vertebra
23–Pedicle of T_{11} vertebra
24–Transverse process of T_{11} vertebra
25–Costotransverse joint
26–Longissimus thoracis
27–Costal tubercle of 11th rib
28–Iliocostalis lumborum muscle

29–Right costodiaphragmatic pleural recess (artifactually enlarged)
30–Serratus posterior inferior muscle
31–Diaphragm
32–Latissimus dorsi muscle
33–Azygous vein
34–Thoracic duct
35–Right suprarenal gland
36–Intercostal muscles
37–Inferior vena cava
38–Caudate lobe of liver
39–Right lobe of liver
40–Falciform ligament

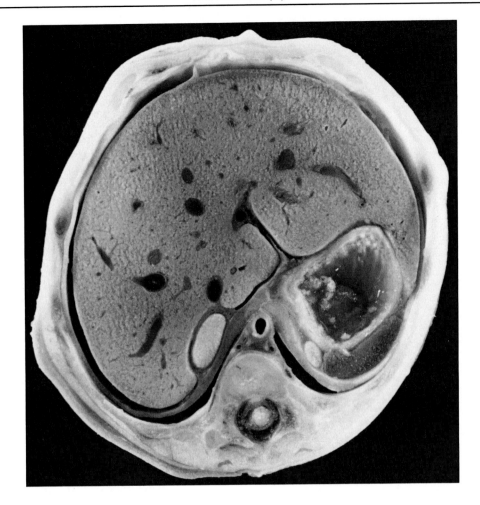

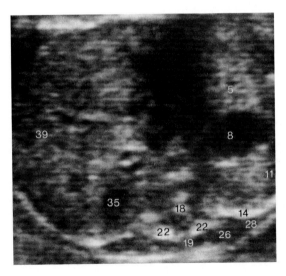

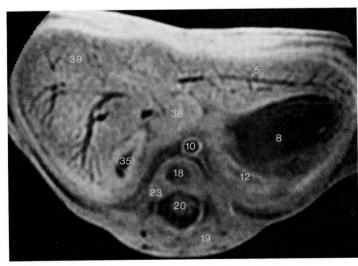

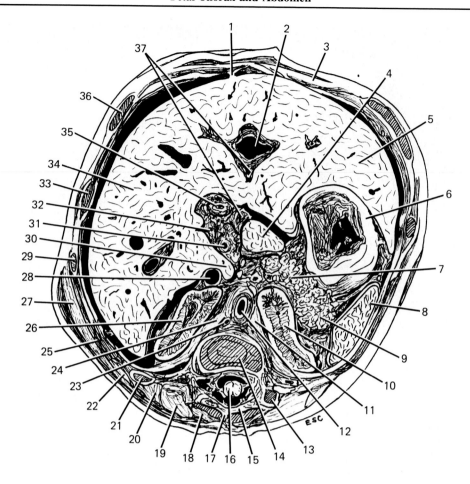

1–Falciform ligament
2–Anastomosis of left branch of
     portal vein and umbilical vein
3–Left rectus abdominis muscle
4–Caudate lobe of liver
5–Left lobe of liver
6–Stomach
7–Body of pancreas
8–Spleen
9–Tail of pancreas
10–Left suprarenal gland
11–Left crus of diaphragm
12–Abdominal aorta
13–Transverse process of L₁ vertebra

14–Body of L₁ vertebra
15–Lamina of L₁ vertebra
16–Spinal medulla (cord)
17–Spinous process
18–Multifidi muscles
19–Longissimus thoracis muscle
20–Iliocostalis lumborum muscle
21–12th rib
22–Origin of internal oblique and
     transverse abdominal muscles
23–Cisterna chyli
24–Right crus of diaphragm
25–11th rib
26–Right suprarenal gland

27–Latissimus dorsi muscle
28–Inferior vena cava
29–10th rib
30–Caudate process of liver
31–Right branch of portal vein
32–Proper hepatic artery
33–9th rib
34–Right lobe of liver
35–Common hepatic duct
36–Costal margin
37–Left branch of portal vein
38–Gallbladder
39–Umbilical vein

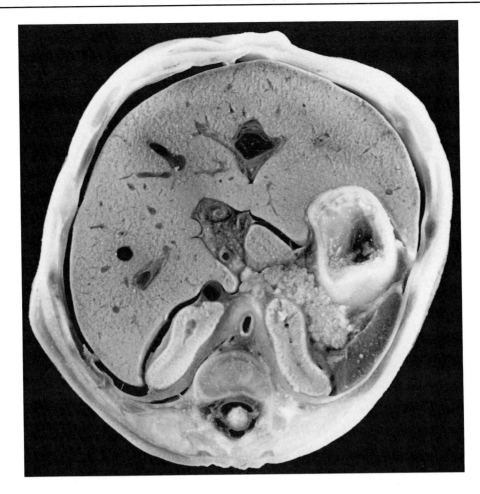

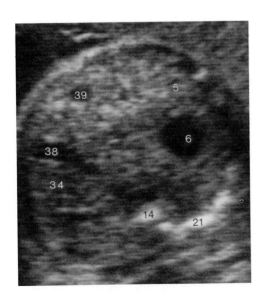

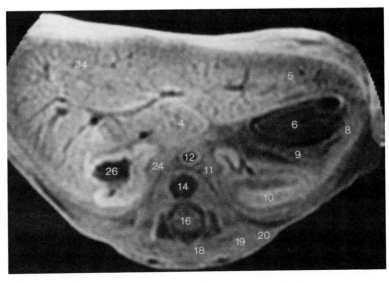

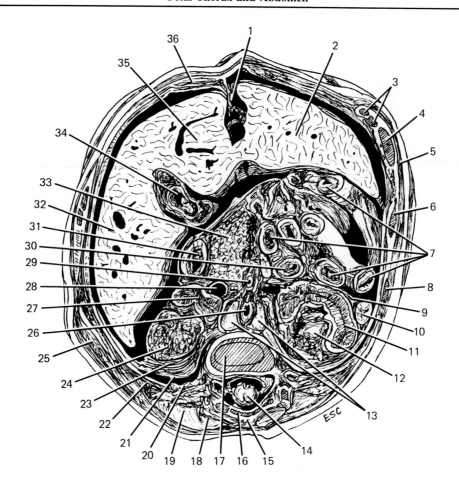

1–Falciform ligament
2–Left lobe of liver
3–Costal margin
4–10th costal cartilage
5–External abdominal oblique muscle
6–11th rib
7–Jejunum
8–12th rib
9–Fused mesocolon and anterior layer of renal fascia
10–Descending colon
11–Left suprarenal gland
12–Left kidney

13–Crura of diaphragm
14–Spinal medulla (cord)
15–Spinous process of L$_2$ vertebra
16–Lamina of L$_2$ vertebra
17–Body of L$_2$ vertebra
18–Multifidi muscles
19–Erector spinae muscle
20–Quadratus lumborum muscle
21–Diaphragm
22–Origin of internal oblique and transverse abdominal muscles from thoracolumbar fascia
23–Pararenal fat body
24–Right kidney

25–Latissimus dorsi
26–Abdominal aorta
27–Right suprarenal gland
28–Inferior vena cava
29–Common bile duct
30–Ascending part of duodenum
31–Descending part of duodenum
32–Right lobe of liver
33–Head of pancreas
34–Body of gall bladder
35–Quadrate lobe of liver
36–Right rectus abdominis muscle

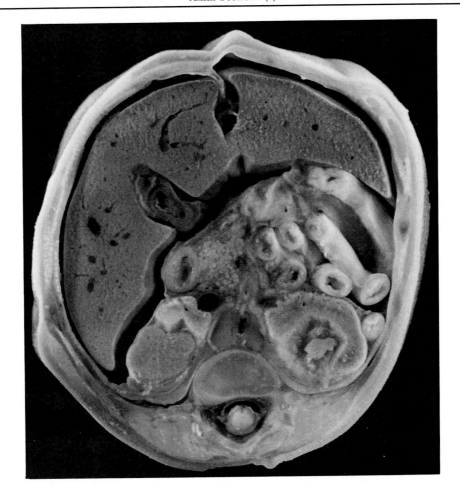

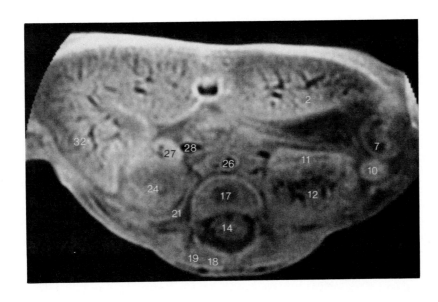

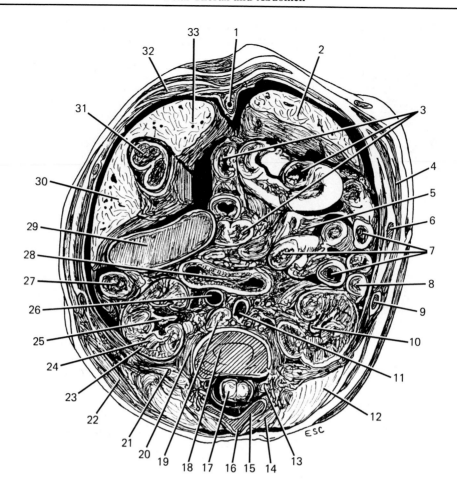

1–Umbilical vein sheathed by
    falciform ligament
2–Left lobe of liver
3–Jejunum
4–External oblique, internal oblique
    and transverse abdominal muscles
5–Mesentery of small intestine
6–11th rib
7–Jejunum
8–Descending colon
9–12th rib
10–Major calyx of left kidney
11–Abdominal aorta
12–Erector spinae muscle

13–Dorsal ganglion of L₃ spinal nerve
14–Multifidi muscles
15–Lamina of L₃ vertebra
16–Spinous process of L₃ vertebra
17–Spinal medulla (cord)
18–Body of L₃ vertebra
19–Right crus of diaphragm
20–Psoas major muscle
21–Quadratus lumborum muscle
22–Latissimus dorsi muscle
23–Cortex of right kidney
24–Medulla of right kidney
25–Pelvis of right kidney
26–Inferior vena cava

27–Ascending colon
28–Inferior or horizontal part of
    duodenum
29–Meconium in transverse colon
30–Right lobe of liver
31–Fundus of gall bladder
32–Right rectus abdominis muscle
33–Quadrate lobe of liver
34–Renal pelvic fat—30 week
    gestation
35–Renal parenchyma
36–Rib

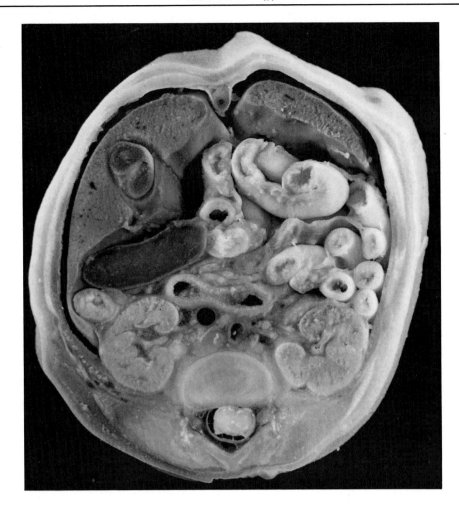

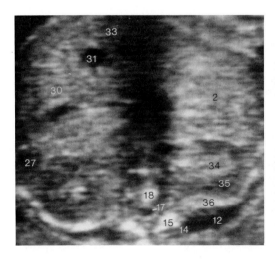

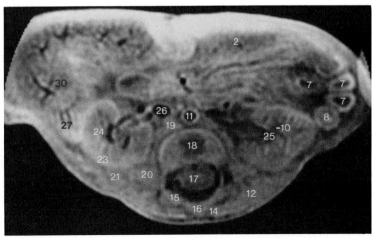

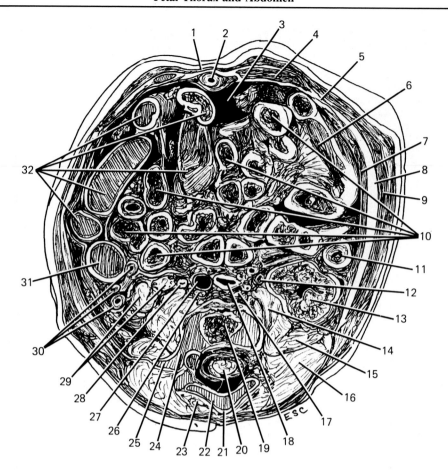

1–Linea alba
2–Umbilical vein
3–Peritoneal cavity
4–Rectus abdominis muscle
5–Semilunar line
6–Mesentery of small intestine
7–Transverse abdominal muscle
8–Internal oblique abdominal muscle
9–External oblique abdominal
    muscle
10–Ileum
11–Descending colon
12–Left ureter

13–Left kidney
14–Psoas major muscle
15–Quadratus lumborum muscle
16–Erector spinae muscle
17–Ganglion of left lumbar
    sympathetic trunk
18–Abdominal aorta
19–Ossification center of body of L$_4$
    vertebra
20–Spinal medulla (cord)
21–Spinous process of L$_4$ vertebra
22–Lamina of L$_4$ vertebra
23–Multifidi muscles

24–Pedicle of L$_4$ vertebra
25–Transverse process of L$_4$ vertebra
26–Ganglion of right lumbar
    sympathetic trunk
27–Inferior vena cava
28–Right ureter
29–Inferior pole of right kidney
30–Vermiform appendix
31–Meconium in ascending colon
32–Meconium in transverse colon
33–Bifurcation of abdominal aorta

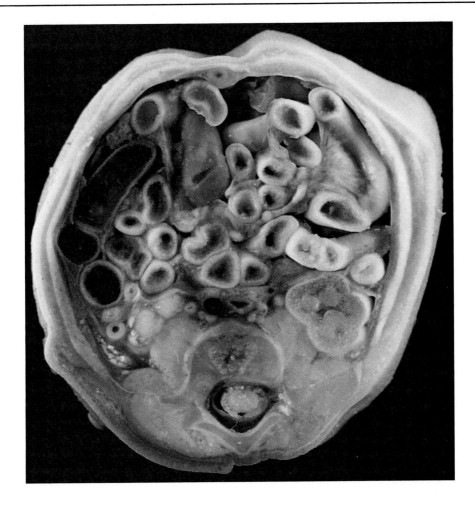

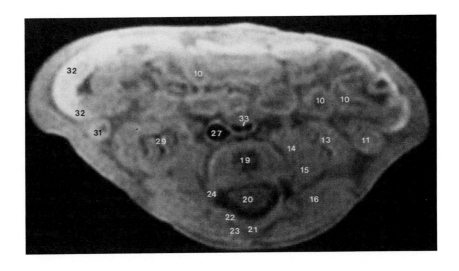

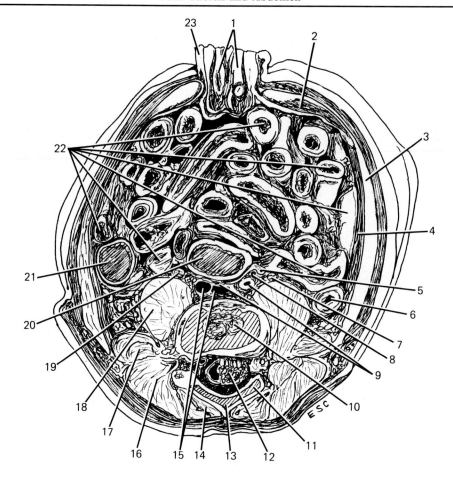

1–Umbilical arteries
2–Rectus abdominis muscle
3–External and internal oblique
   abdominal muscles
4–Transverse abdominal muscle
5–Superior rectal artery
6–Descending colon
7–Left ureter
8–Superior rectal vein

9–Common iliac arteries
10–Ossification center of body of L$_5$
   vertebra
11–Lamina of L$_5$ vertebra
12–Cauda equina (Dorsal and ventral
   roots of S$_{1–5}$, and coccygeal spinal
   nerves)
13–Spinous process of L$_5$ vertebra
14–Multifidi muscles

15–Common iliac veins
16–Erector spinae muscle
17–Quadratus lumborum muscle
18–Psoas major muscle
19–Right ureter
20–Meconium in rectum
21–Meconium in cecum
22–Ileum
23–Stump of umbilical cord

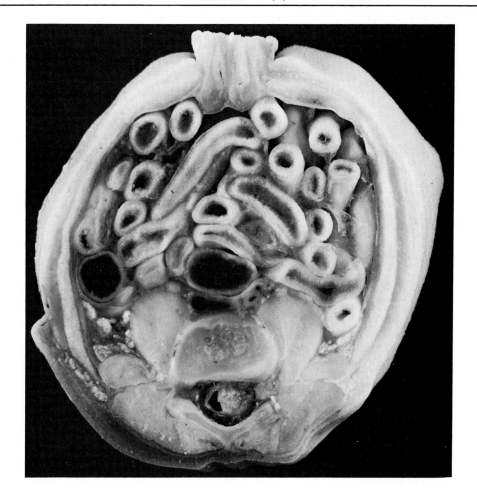

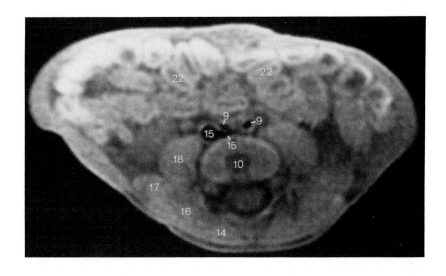

Fetal Thorax and Abdomen

SECTION 1

Axial Sections

20 Week Fetus

Male Pelvis

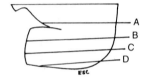

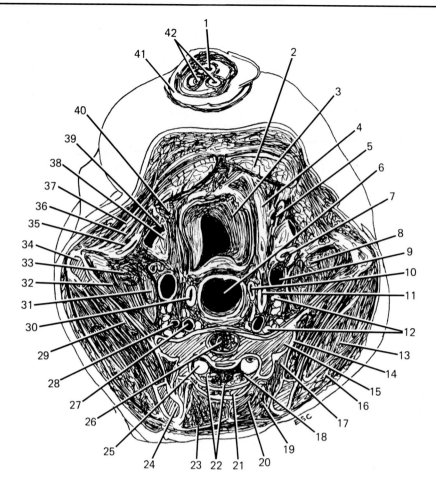

1–Umbilical vein
2–Rectus abdominis muscle
3–Body of urinary bladder
4–Left umbilical artery
5–Left umbilical vein
6–Rectum
7–External iliac artery
8–Left femoral nerve
9–External iliac vein
10–Left ureter
11–Lumen of left umbilical artery
12–Sacral plexus nerves
13–Gluteus medius muscle
14–Sacroiliac joint
15–Lateral part of sacrum
16–Gluteus maximus muscle
17–Interosseous sacroiliac ligament

18–Sacral canal
19–Erector spinae muscle
20–Multifidi muscles
21–Dorsal part of sacrum
22–Cauda equina
23–Posterior layer of thoracolumbar
   fascia
24–Posterior superior iliac spine
25–S₂ spinal nerve
26–Ossification center of base of 2nd
   vertebral segment of sacrum
27–Internal iliac vein
28–Internal iliac artery
29–Ala of ilium
30–Right ureter
31–Psoas major part of iliopsoas
   muscle

32–Iliacus part of iliopsoas muscle
33–Right femoral nerve
34–Anterior superior iliac spine
35–Transverse abdominal muscle
36–Internal oblique abdominal muscle
37–External oblique abdominal
   muscle
38–Gubernaculum
39–Processus vaginalis
40–Right umbilical artery
41–Stump of umbilical cord
42–Umbilical arteries
43–Sacral ossification center

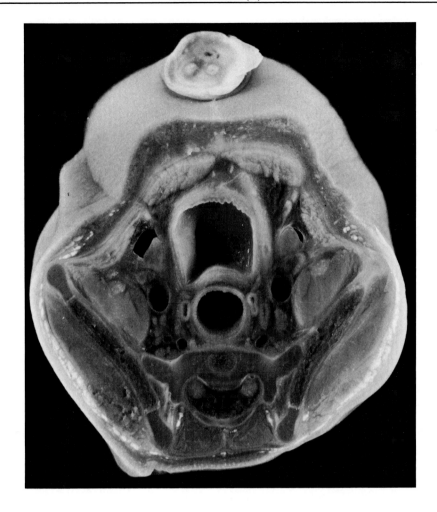

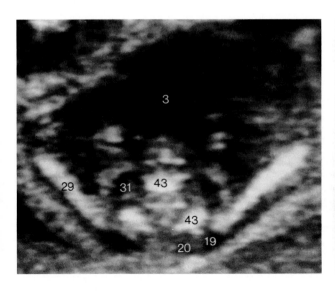

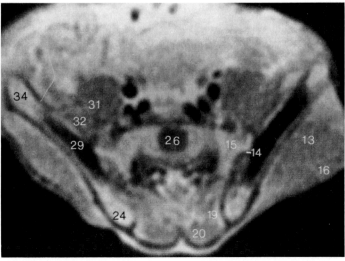

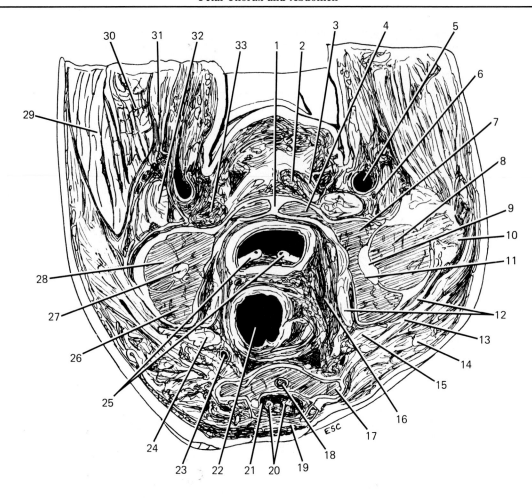

1–Pubic symphysis
2–Rectus femoris
3–Falx inguinalis (conjoined tendon)
4–Superior ramus of pubis
5–Femoral vein
6–Femoral artery
7–Body of pubis
8–Head of left femur
9–Ligament of head of left femur
10–Greater trochanter of femur
11–Acetabulum of hip joint
12–Internal obturator muscle
13–Gluteus medius muscle
14–Gluteus maximus muscle
15–Left sciatic nerve
16–Levator ani muscle
17–Lateral part of sacrum
18–Ossification center of base of 5th
    vertebral segment of sacrum
19–Superficial dorsal sacrococcygeal
    ligament covering sacral hiatus
20–Cauda equina (roots of coccygeal
    spinal nerves)
21–Sacral canal
22–Rectum
23–Inferior gluteal vein
24–Right sciatic nerve
25–Ureter opening into urinary
    bladder
26–Body of ischium
27–Ligament of head of right femur
28–Head of right femur
29–Tensor fasciae latae muscle
30–Sartorius muscle
31–Rectus femoris muscle
32–Iliopsoas muscle
33–Pectineus muscle
34–Ischial ossification center
35–Proximal femur

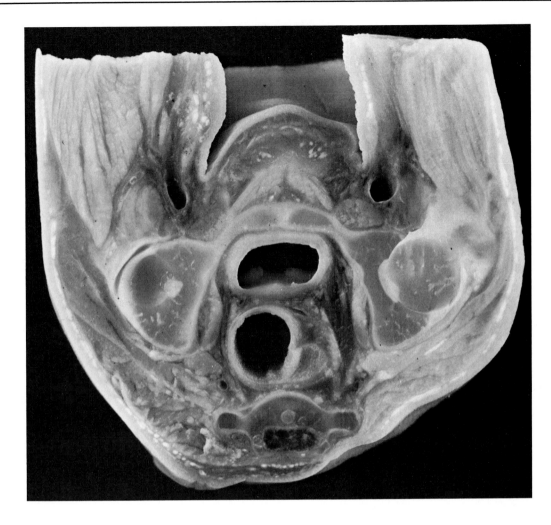

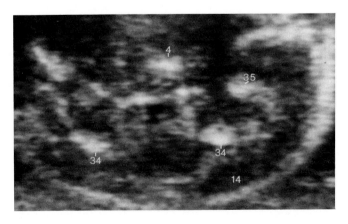

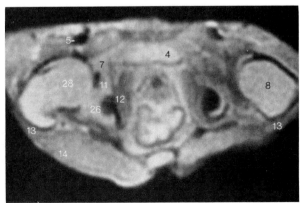

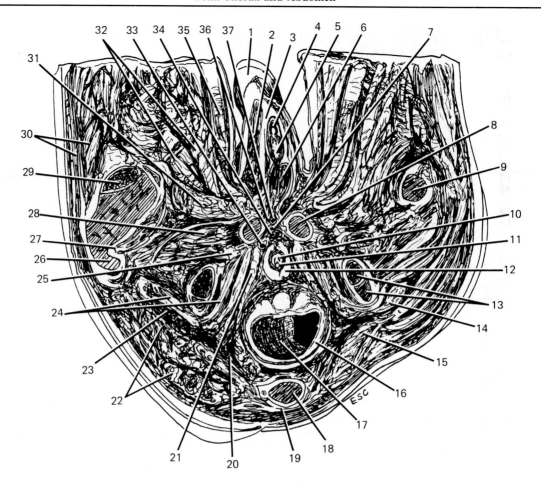

1–Penis
2–Corpus cavernosum penis
3–Tunica albuginea
4–Corpus spongiosum penis
5–Penile urethra
6–Bulb of corpus spongiosum penis
7–Arcuate pubic ligament
8–Left pubis
9–Dorsal projection of upper shaft of
    femur
10–Prostatic urethra
11–Prostatic utricle
12–Prostate gland
13–Ossified and cartilagenous parts of
    left ischial tuberosity

14–Left sciatic nerve
15–Ischiorectal fossa fat
16–Rectum
17–Transverse rectal fold
18–1st vertebral segment of coccyx
19–Deep dorsal sacrococcygeal
    ligament
20–Piriformis muscle
21–Levator ani muscle
22–Gluteus maximus muscle
23–Right sciatic nerve
24–Obturator internus muscle
25–Obturator membrane
26–Intertrochanteric crest
27–Trochanteric fossa

28–Obturator externus muscle
29–Ossified part of upper shaft of
    femur
30–Vastus lateralis muscle
31–Adductor magnus muscle
32–Adductor brevis muscle
33–Right internal pudendal vein
34–Right internal pudendal artery
35–Adductor longus muscle
36–Dorsal nerve of penis
37–Dorsal artery of penis
38–Ossified portion of right ischial
    tuberosity

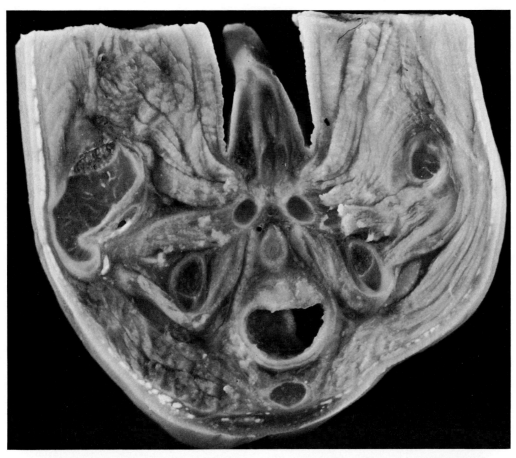

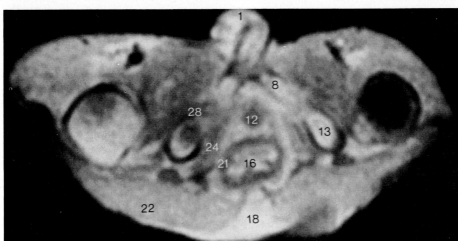

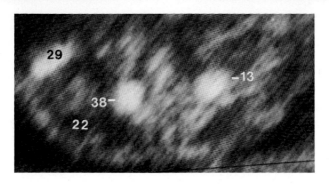

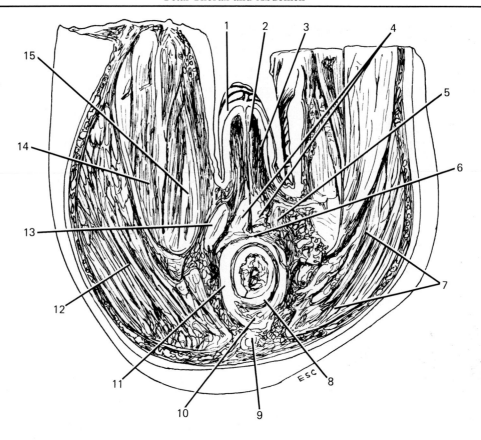

1–Scrotum
2–Scrotal septum
3–Dartos tunic
4–Bulbospongiosus muscle
5–Left ischiocavernosus muscle
6–Central perineal tendon
7–Left gluteus maximus muscle
8–Internal anal sphincter

9–Distal tip of coccyx
10–Anococcygeal ligament
11–External anal sphincter muscle
12–Right gluteus maximus muscle
13–Right ischiocavernosus muscle
14–Long head of biceps femoris
   muscle

15–Semitendinosus muscle
16–Penis
17–Descended testis—30 week
   gestation
18–Proximal shaft of femur
19–Anus

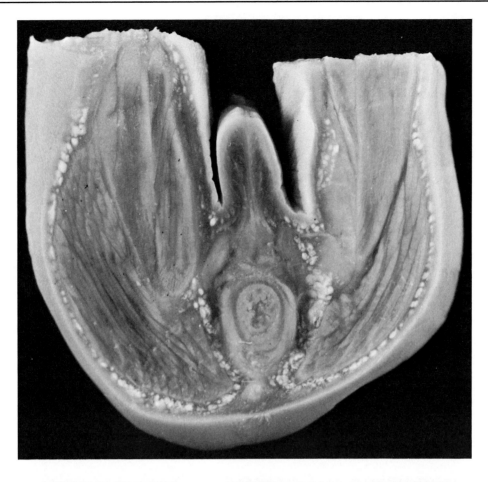

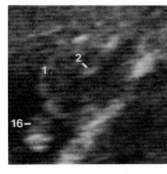

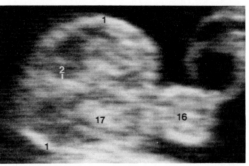

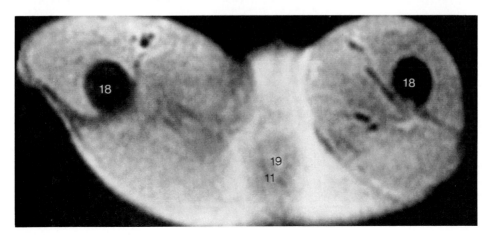

Fetal Thorax and Abdomen

SECTION 1

Axial Sections

20 Week Fetus

Female Pelvis

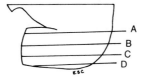

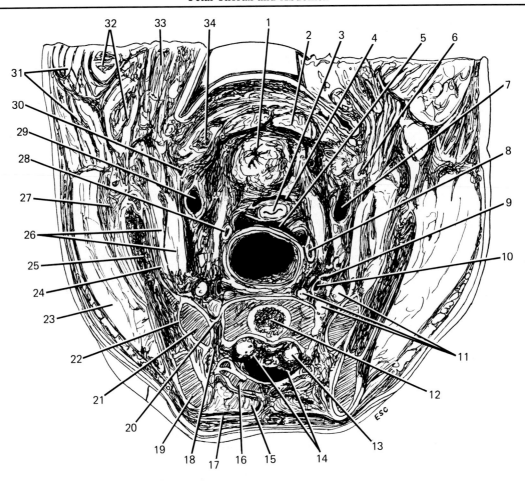

1–Body of contracted urinary
   bladder
2–Rectus abdominis muscle
3–Body of uterus
4–Vesicouterine pouch
5–Rectouterine pouch
6–Left external iliac artery
7–Left external iliace vein
8–Left ureter
9–Internal iliac artery
10–Internal iliac vein
11–Sacral plexus nerves
12–Ossification center of base of S₂
   vertebral segment of sacrum
13–S₂ spinal nerve
14–Cauda equina
15–Erector spinae and multifidi
   muscles
16–Dorsal part of sacrum
17–Posterior layer of thoracolumbar
   fascia
18–Posterior sacral foramen
19–Posterior superior iliac spine
20–Anterior sacral foramen
21–Lateral part of sacrum
22–Sacroiliac joint
23–Gluteus maximus muscle
24–Iliac fossa
25–Ala of ilium
26–Iliopsoas muscle
27–Gluteus medius muscle
28–Right ureter
29–Right external iliac vein
30–Right external iliac artery
31–Tensor fasciae latae muscle
32–Sartorius muscle
33–Rectus femoris muscle
34–Round ligament of uterus at right
   inguinal ring

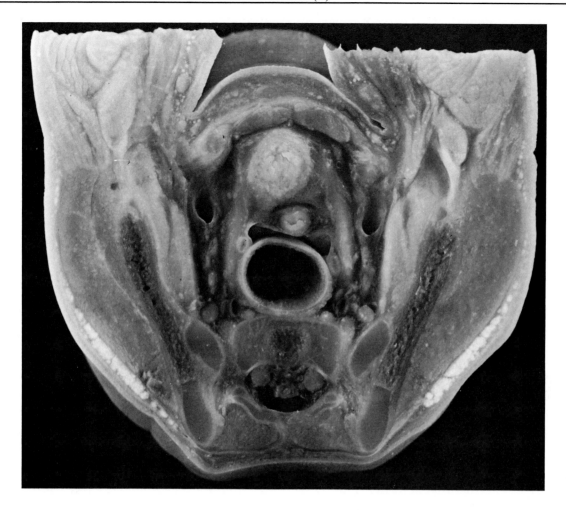

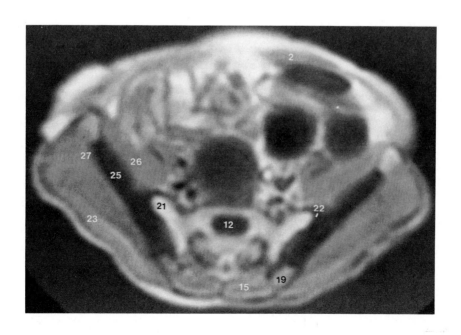

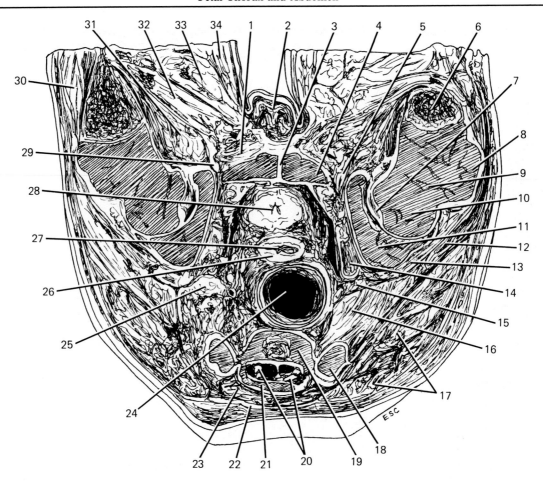

1–Pectineus muscle
2–Anterior labial commissure
3–Pubic symphysis
4–Superior ramus of left pubis
5–Left obturator nerve passing
through obturator canal
6–Ossified upper shaft (metaphysis)
of femur
7–Ligament of head of femur
8–Greater trochanter
9–Neck of femur
10–Head of femur
11–Body of ischium
12–Gluteus medius and minimus
muscles

13–Superior gemellus muscle
14–Obturator internus muscle
15–Left sciatic nerve
16–Piriformis muscle
17–Gluteus maximus muscle
18–Lateral part of sacrum
19–Base of S₃ vertebral segment of
sacrum
20–Cauda equina
21–Dorsal part of sacrum
22–Posterior layer of thoracolumbar
fascia
23–Erector spinae and multifidi
muscles
24–Rectum

25–Right sciatic nerve
26–Vagina
27–Cervix of uterus
28–Urethral opening of urinary
bladder
29–Right obturator nerve
30–Tensor fasciae latae muscle
31–Adductor magnus muscle
32–Adductor brevis muscle
33–Adductor longus muscle
34–Gracilis muscle

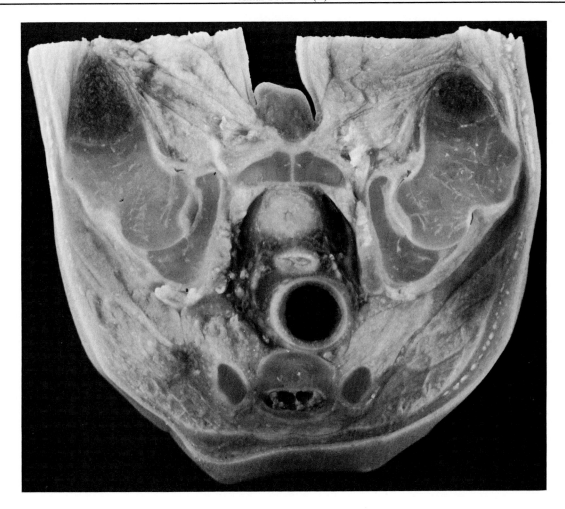

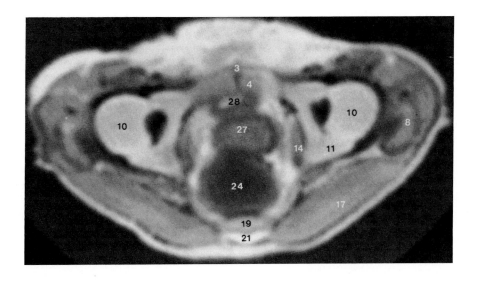

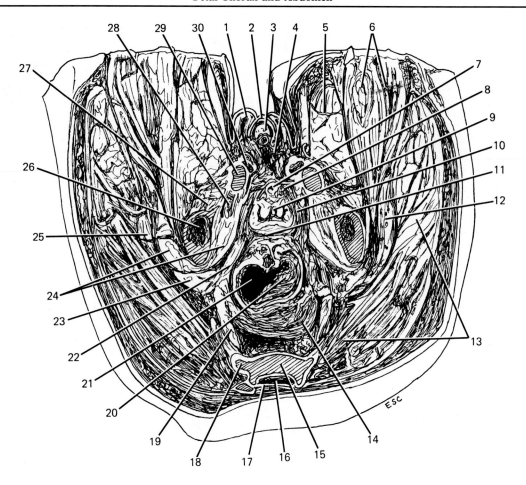

1–Right labium majus
2–Prepuce of clitoris
3–Glans of clitoris
4–Left labium minus
5–Semitendinosus muscle
6–Long head of biceps femoris
   muscle
7–Membranous urethra
8–Sphincter urethrae muscle of
   urogenital diaphragm
9–Vagina lined with cornified
   epithelium
10–Vaginal sphincter muscle of
   urogenital diaphragm

11–Central perineal tendon (perineal
   body)
12–Left sciatic nerve
13–Gluteus maximus muscle
14–Levator ani muscle
15–Base of S₅ vertebral segment of
   sacrum
16–Sacral hiatus
17–Posterior deep sacrococcygeal
   ligament
18–Lateral part of sacrum
19–Sacrotuberous ligament
20–Transverse rectal fold
21–Rectum

22–Levator ani muscle
23–Sacrotuberous ligament
24–Obturator internus muscle
25–Right sciatic nerve
26–Ischial tuberosity
27–Obturator externus muscle
28–Obturator membrane
29–Inferior ramus of right pubis
30–Right crus of clitoris
31–Right labrum minus
32–Left labrum majus
33–Proximal thigh

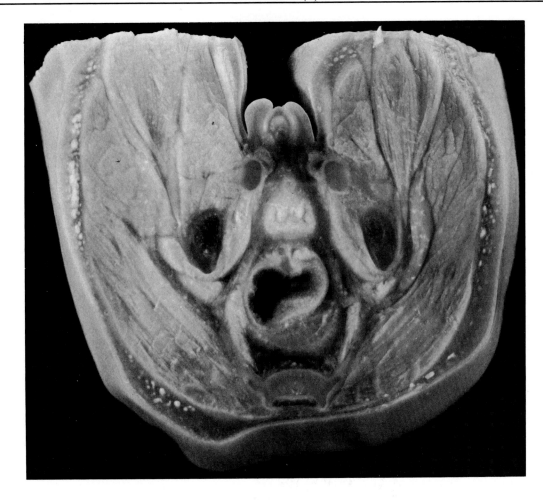

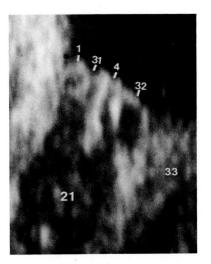

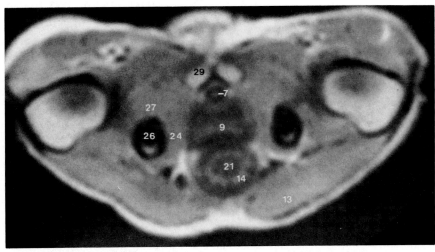

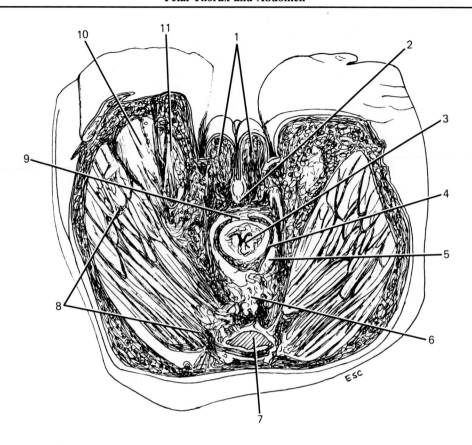

1–Labia majora
2–Posterior labial commissure
3–Anal canal
4–Internal anal sphincter muscle
5–External anal sphincter muscle

6–Anococcygeal ligament
7–Coccyx
8–Gluteus maximus muscle
9–Central perineal tendon (perineal body)

10–Long head of biceps femoris muscle
11–Semitendinosus muscle
12–Proximal femoral shaft

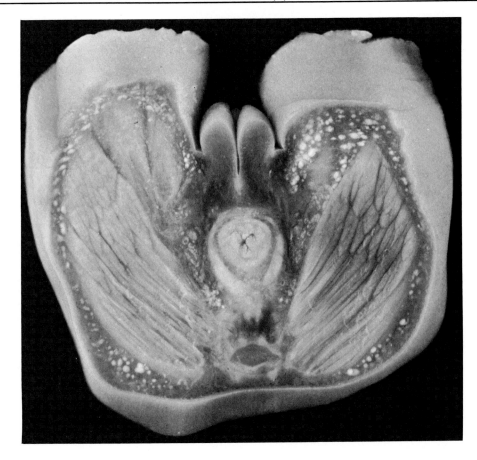

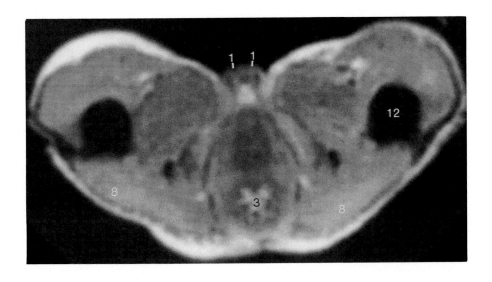

Fetal Thorax and Abdomen

SECTION 2

Sagittal Sections

20 Week Fetus

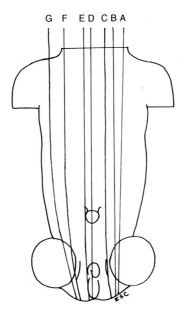

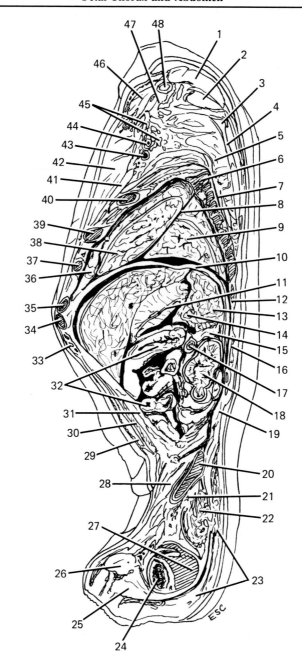

1–Trapezius muscle
2–Supraspinatus muscle
3–Spine of scapula
4–Body of scapula
5–Subscapularis muscle
6–2nd rib
7–Serratus anterior muscle
8–Oblique fissure
9–Inferior lobe of left lung

10–Diaphragm
11–Greater curvature of stomach
12–11th rib
13–Spleen
14–Tail of pancreas
15–Left suprarenal gland
16–12th rib
17–Left flexure (splenic) of colon
18–Left kidney

19–Latissimus dorsi muscle
20–Ala of ilium
21–Gluteus minimus muscle
22–Gluteus medius muscle
23–Gluteus maximus muscle
24–Ossified upper shaft of left femur
25–Vastus lateralis muscle
26–Rectus femoris muscle
27–Greater trochanter of femur

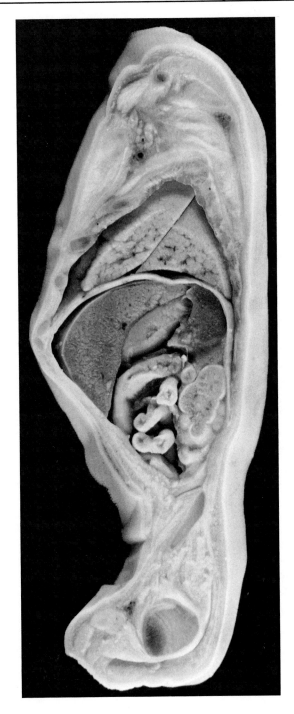

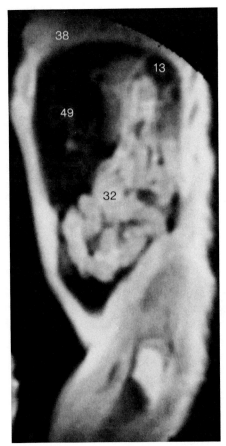

28–Iliopsoas muscle
29–External oblique abdominal
    muscle
30–Internal oblique abdominal muscle
31–Transverse abdominal muscle
32–Jejunum
33–Costal angle
34–6th costal cartilage
35–5th costal cartilage

36–Apex of heart
37–4th costal cartilage
38–Lingula of superior lobe of left
    lung
39–3rd rib
40–2nd rib
41–Pectoralis minor muscle
42–Sternal part of pectoralis major
    muscle

43–Axillary vein
44–Axillary artery
45–Nerves from brachial plexus to left
    upper limb
46–Clavicular part of pectoralis major
    muscle
47–Subclavius muscle
48–Clavicle
49–Left lobe of liver

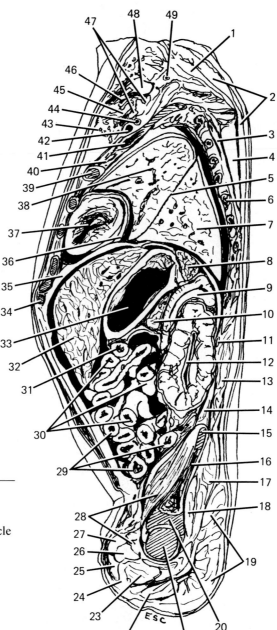

1–Levator scapulae muscle
2–Trapezius muscle
3–Serratus posterior superior muscle
4–Rhomboideus major muscle
5–Oblique fissure
6–6th rib
7–Inferior lobe of left lung
8–Spleen
9–Left suprarenal gland
10–Body of pancreas
11–12th rib
12–Pelvis of left kidney
13–Erector spinae muscle
14–Quadratus lumborum muscle
15–Crest of ilium
16–Ala of ilium
17–Gluteus medius muscle
18–Gluteus minimus muscle
19–Gluteus maximus muscle
20–Acetabulum
21–Head of femur
22–Semitendinosus muscle
23–Adductor magnus muscle
24–Adductor brevis muscle
25–Adductor longus muscle
26–Obturator externus muscle

27–Pectineus muscle
28–Iliopsoas muscle
29–Ileum
30–Jejunum
31–Transverse colon
32–Left lobe of liver
33–Body of stomach
34–7th costal cartilage
35–Diaphragm

36–Pericardium
37–Left ventricle
38–Superior lobe of left lung
39–2nd costal cartilage
40–Internal intercostal muscle
41–1st rib
42–Subclavian vein
43–Pectoralis major muscle
44–Subclavian artery

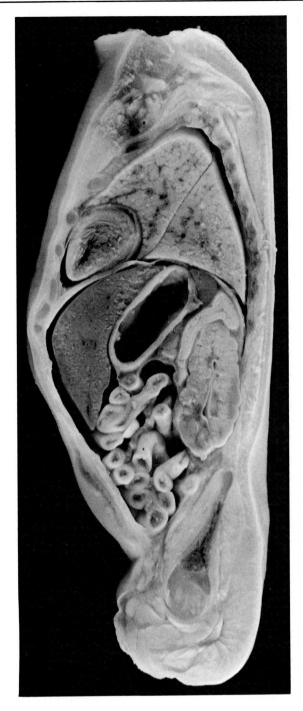

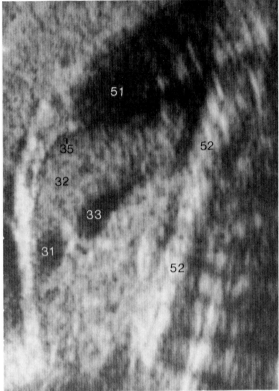

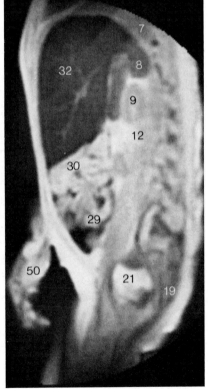

45–Subclavius muscle
46–Clavicle
47–Nerves from brachial plexus to left
    upper limb
48–Inferior belly of omohyoid muscle
49–Transverse cervical artery
50–Hand
51–Thorax
52–Spine

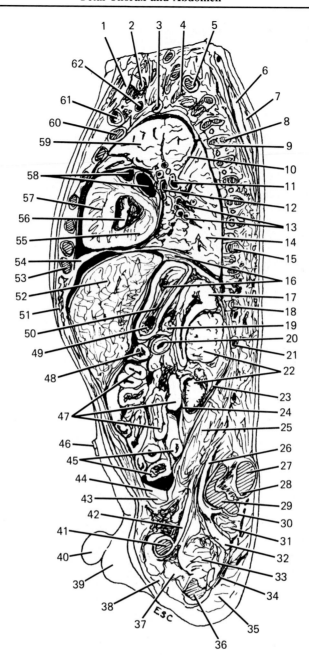

1–Sternohyoid muscle
2–Inferior belly of omohyoid muscle
3–Subclavian artery
4–Head of 1st rib
5–Body of T_1 vertebra
6–Splenius capitis muscle
7–Trapezius muscle
8–Body of T_4 vertebra
9–Head of 4th rib
10–Oblique fissure
11–Left main bronchus
12–Left pulmonary artery
13–Left pulmonary veins

14–Inferior lobe of left lung
15–9th rib
16–Esophagus
17–Left suprarenal gland
18–11th rib
19–Neck of pancreas
20–Inferior or horizontal part of
   duodenum
21–12th rib
22–Left kidney
23–Posterior layer of renal fascia
24–Anterior layer of renal fascia
25–Psoas major muscle

26–Left lumbosacral nerve trunk
27–Tuberosity of ilium
28–Posterior superior iliac spine
29–Auricular (articular) surface of
   ilium
30–Posterior inferior iliac spine
31–Piriformis muscle
32–Sciatic nerve
33–Left levator ani muscle
34–Sacrotuberous ligament
35–Gluteus maximus muscle
36–Ischial tuberosity
37–Obturator internus muscle

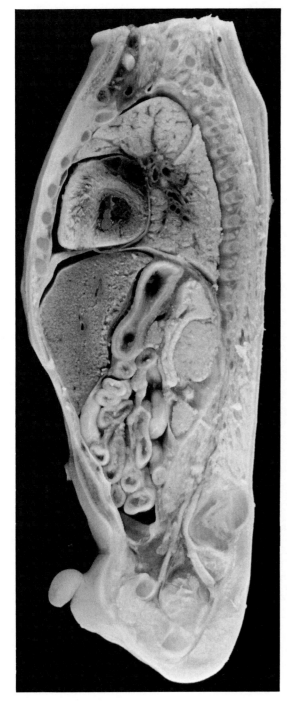

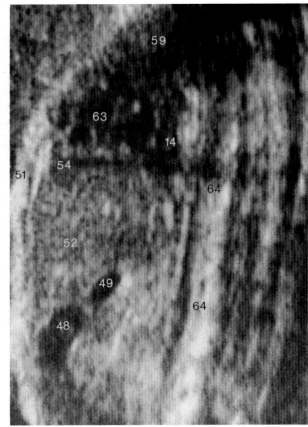

38–Obturator externus muscle
39–Left side of scrotum
40–Penis
41–Superior ramus of left pubis
42–Left obturator nerve
43–Urinary bladder
44–Left umbilical artery
45–Ileum
46–Stump of umbilical cord

47–Jejunum
48–Transverse colon
49–Pylorus
50–Lesser curvature of stomach
51–Costal angle
52–Left lobe of liver
53–7th costal cartilage
54–Diaphragm
55–Left ventricle

56–Papillary muscle
57–Right ventricle
58–Left atrium
59–Superior lobe of left lung
60–1st costal cartilage
61–Clavicle
62–Subclavian vein
63–Heart
64–Spine

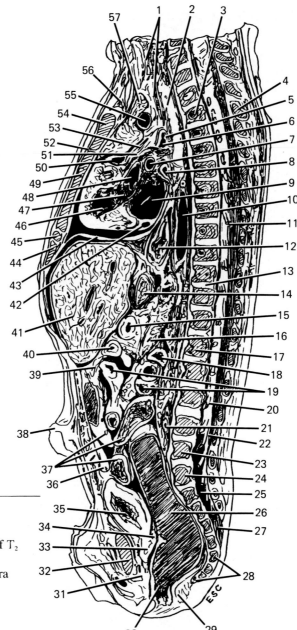

1–Trachea
2–Esophagus
3–Ossification center of body of T_2 vertebra
4–Spinous process of T_2 vertebra
5–Lumen of arch of aorta
6–Lumen of ductus arteriosus
7–Left pulmonary artery
8–Left main bronchus
9–Left atrium
10–Descending thoracic aorta
11–Left T_7 spinal nerve roots
12–Cardiac orifice of stomach
13–Intervertebral disc between bodies of T_{10} and T_{11} vertebrae
14–Caudate lobe of liver
15–Pylorus of stomach
16–Head of pancreas
17–Body of T_{12} vertebra
18–Inferior or horizontal part of duodenum
19–Jejunum
20–Dura mater enclosing caudal extent of spinal medulla (cord) in vertebral canal

21–Left common iliac artery
22–Dura mater enclosing cauda equina
23–Body of L_5 vertebra
24–1st vertebral segment of base of sacrum
25–Sacral canal
26–Meconium filled rectum

27–Sacral hiatus
28–Coccyx
29–External anal sphincter muscle
30–Anal canal
31–Urogenital diaphragm
32–Left pubis
33–Prostate gland
34–Left seminal vesicle

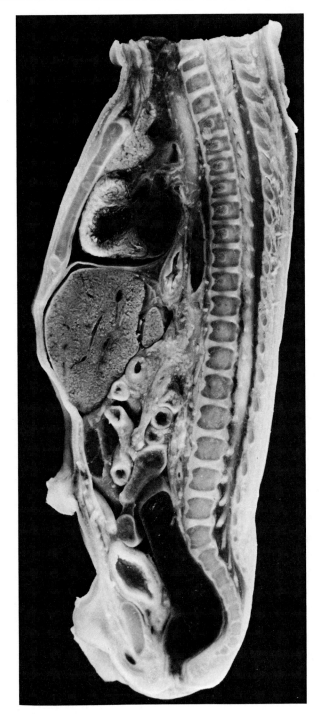

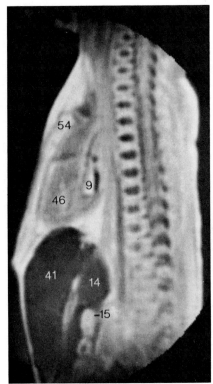

35–Urinary bladder
36–Left umbilical artery
37–Sigmoid colon
38–Stump of umbilical cord
39–Lesser omentum
40–Transverse colon
41–Left lobe of liver
42–Coronary sinus

43–Diaphragm
44–Xiphoid process of sternum
45–Left 7th costal cartilage
46–Right ventricle
47–Membranous part of
    interventricular septum
48–Ascending aorta
49–Body of sternum

50–Appendage of right atrium
51–Pulmonary trunk
52–Sternal angle
53–Ductus arteriosus
54–Manubrium of sternum
55–Left brachiocephalic vein
56–Suprasternal fascial space
57–Thymus gland

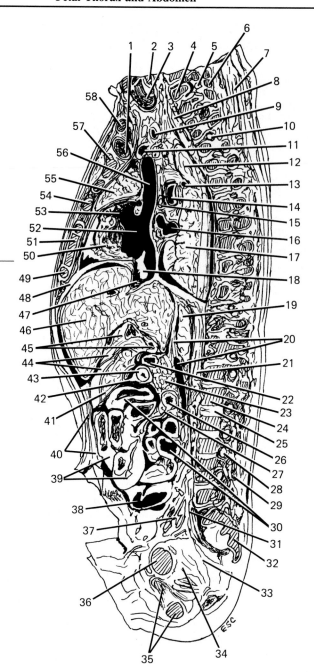

1–Right clavicle
2–Cricoid cartilage
3–Trachea
4–Body of C$_5$ vertebra
5–Right C$_5$ spinal nerve
6–Spinous process of C$_5$ vertebra
7–Ligamentum nuchae
8–Right longus colli muscle
9–Brachiocephalic artery
10–Right C$_8$ spinal nerve
11–Right brachiocephalic vein
12–Superior lobe of right lung
13–Azygos vein
14–Right main bronchus
15–Right pulmonary artery
16–Right pulmonary vein
17–Inferior lobe of right lung
18–Clot in inferior vena cava
19–Right suprarenal gland
20–Inferior vena cava
21–Right crus of diaphragm
22–Superior part of duodenum
23–Head of pancreas
24–Body of L$_1$ vertebra
25–Intervertebral disc
26–Inferior or horizontal part of
    duodenum
27–Mesentery of small intestine
28–Right L$_2$ spinal nerve
29–Spinous process of L$_2$ vertebra
30–Jejunum
31–Right lumbosacral nerve trunk
32–Auricular (articular) surface of
    lateral part of sacrum
33–Coccygeus muscle
34–Right levator ani muscle
35–Inferior ramus of pubis
36–Superior ramus of pubis
37–Psoas major muscle
38–Sigmoid colon
39–Ileum
40–Extrahepatic umbilical vein

41–Quadrate lobe of liver
42–Greater omentum
43–Transverse colon
44–Intrahepatic umbilical vein
45–Left branch of portal vein
46–Right lobe of liver
47–Ductus venosus
48–Diaphragm

49–Right 7th costal cartilage
50–Right ventricular wall
51–Sternebra of body of sternum
52–Right atrioventricular opening of
    right atrium
53–Appendage of right atrium
54–Right 3rd costal cartilage
55–Thymus gland

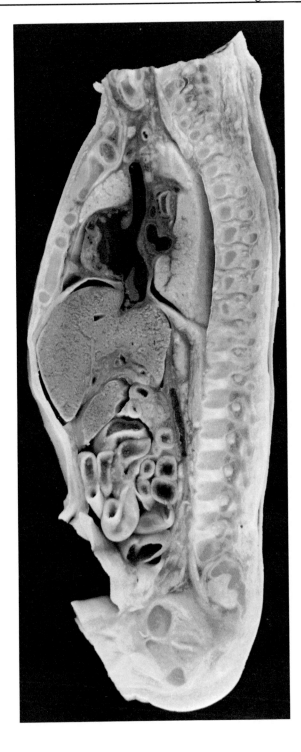

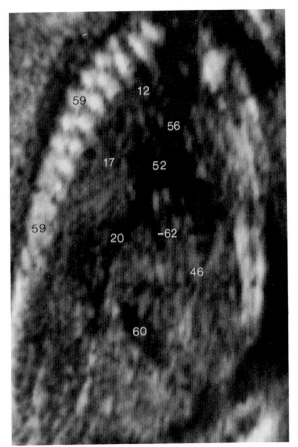

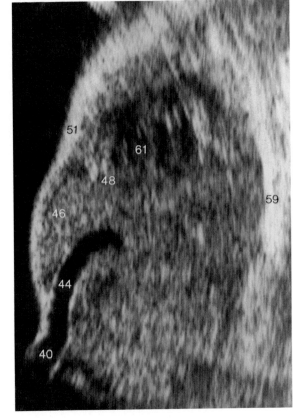

56–Superior vena cava
57–Manubrium of sternum
58–Sternal head of
    sternocleidomastoid muscle
59–Spine
60–Gallbladder
61–Heart
62–Hepatic vein

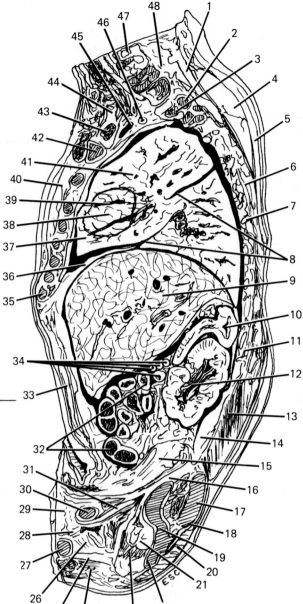

1–Splenius capitis muscle
2–T$_1$ vertebra
3–1st right rib
4–Rhomboideus major muscle
5–Trapezius muscle
6–Longissimus thoracis muscle
7–6th right rib
8–Oblique fissure
9–Right lobe of liver
10–Right suprarenal gland
11–Right 11th rib
12–Pelvis of kidney
13–Erector spinae muscle
14–Quadratus lumborum muscle
15–Psoas major muscle
16–Right lumbosacral nerve trunk
17–Tuberosity of right ilium
18–Posterior superior iliac spine
19–Auricular (articular) surface of
    right ilium
20–Gluteus maximus muscle
21–Piriformis muscle
22–Posterior inferior iliac spine
23–Coccygeus muscle
24–Levator ani muscle
25–Arcus tendineus
26–Obturator internus muscle
27–Inferior ramus of right pubis
28–Obturator externus muscle
29–Pectineus muscle
30–Superior ramus of right pubis

31–Obturator nerve
32–Ileum
33–Right rectus abdominis muscle
34–Vermiform appendix
35–Right 8th costal cartilage
36–Diaphragm
37–Middle lobe of right lung
38–Cardiac impression

39–Transverse fissure
40–Pectoralis major muscle
41–Superior lobe of right lung
42–Right 1st costal cartilage
43–Clavicle
44–Sternocleidomastoid muscle
45–Right subclavian vein
46–Right subclavian artery

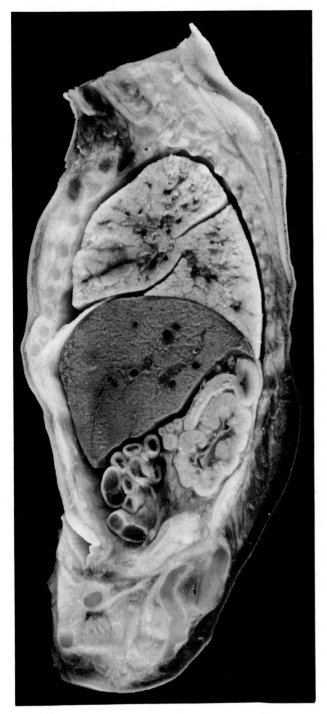

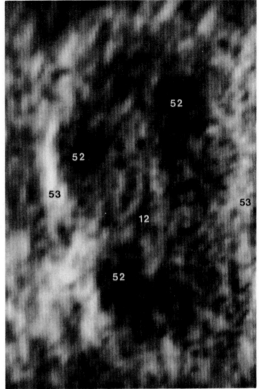

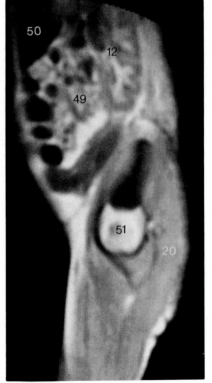

47–Right C$_4$ spinal nerve
48–Semispinalis capitis muscle
49–Small bowel loops
50–Liver
51–Head of femur
52–Renal pyramid—30 week gestation
53–Perinephric capsule/fat

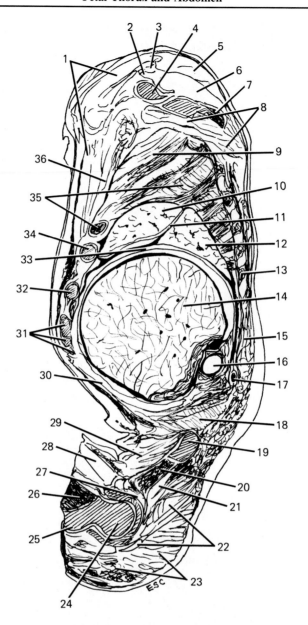

1–Pectoralis major muscle
2–Coracoclavicular ligament
3–Clavicle
4–Coracoid process of right scapula
5–Trapezius muscle
6–Supraspinatus muscle
7–Spine of right scapula
8–Serratus anterior muscle
9–1st rib
10–Middle lobe of right lung
11–Oblique fissure
12–Inferior lobe of right lung
13–9th rib

14–Right lobe of liver
15–Iliocostalis lumborum muscle
16–Lobule of lateral-most surface of
　　right kidney
17–12th rib
18–Internal oblique abdominal muscle
19–Crest of ilium
20–Ala of right ilium
21–Gluteus minimus muscle
22–Gluteus medius muscle
23–Gluteus maximus muscle
24–Head of right femur
25–Greater trochanter

26–Ossified upper shaft of right femur
27–Acetabulum
28–Rectus femoris muscle
29–Iliacus muscle
30–Right costal margin
31–6th–8th costal cartilages
32–5th costal cartilage
33–Diaphragm
34–4th costal cartilage
35–3rd rib
36–Pectoralis minor muscle
37–Gallbladder
38–Spine

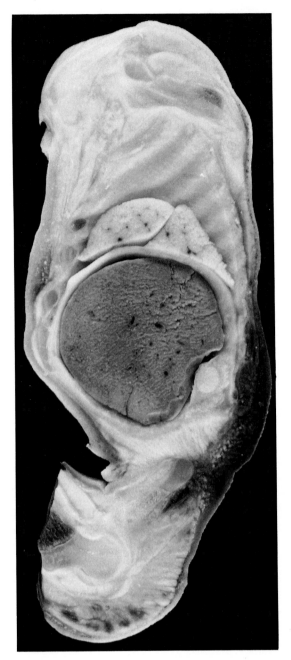

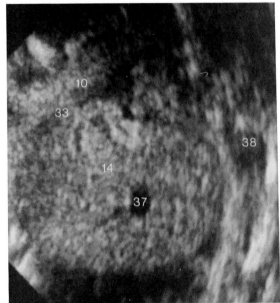

Fetal Thorax and Abdomen

SECTION 3

Coronal Sections

20 Week Fetus

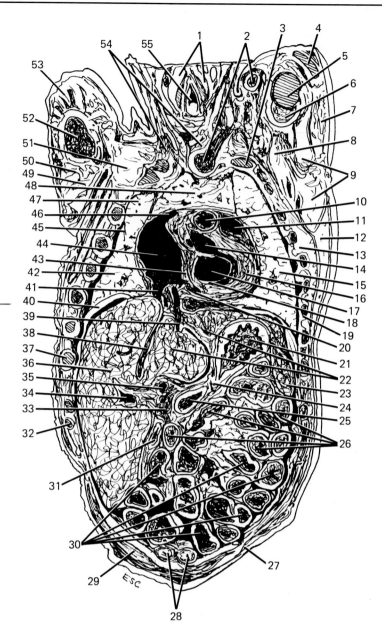

1–Thyroid cartilage
2–Left clavicle
3–Left 1st costal cartilage
4–Acromion
5–Head of left humerus
6–Glenoid cavity
7–Left deltoid muscle
8–Subscapularis muscle
9–Left teres major muscle
10–Pulmonary trunk
11–Appendage of left atrium
12–Latissimus dorsi muscle
13–Left serratus anterior muscle
14–Aortic outflow tract of left
      ventricle
15–Superior lobe of left lung
16–Left ventricular wall
17–Left atrioventricular opening
18–Left fibrous ring of cardiac
      skeleton
19–Left 7th rib
20–Coronary sinus opening
21–Fundus of stomach
22–Left lobe of liver
23–Spleen
24–Lesser curvature of stomach
25–Pyloric antrum of stomach
26–Jejunum
27–Left semilunar line
28–Right and left umbilical arteries
29–Right rectus abdominis muscle
30–Ileum
31–Common bile duct
32–Right 9th costal cartilage
33–Portal vein
34–Right branch of portal vein
35–Left branch of portal vein
36–Right lobe of liver
37–Right 7th costal cartilage

38–Right hepatic vein
39–Ductus venosus
40–Diaphragm
41–Inferior vena cava
42–Middle lobe of right lung
43–Right fibrous trigone of cardiac
      skeleton

44–Left atrium
45–Horizontal fissure
46–Appendage of right atrium
47–Superior lobe of right lung
48–Thymus gland
49–Right teres major muscle
50–Triceps brachii muscle

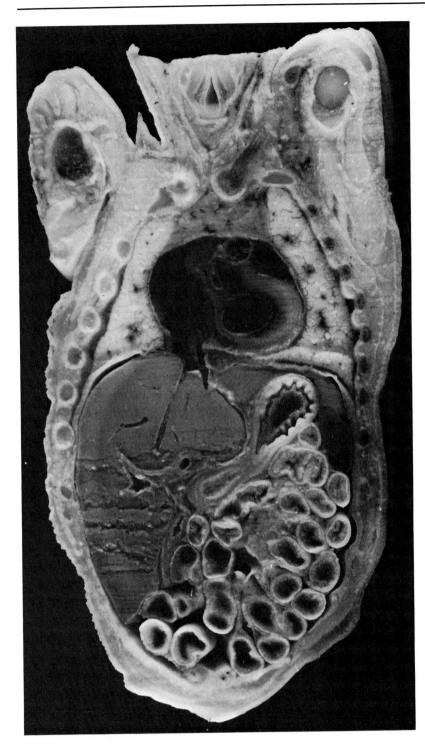

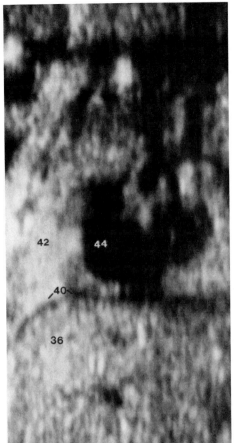

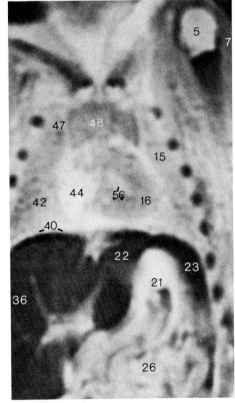

51–Right serratus anterior muscle
52–Ossified upper shaft of humerus
53–Right deltoid muscle
54–Right and left sternocleidomastoid
    muscles
55–Infraglottic cavity of larynx
56–Left ventricular cavity

1–Trachea
2–Body of C₆ vertebra
3–Upper esophagus
4–Left brachiocephalic vein
5–Subscapularis muscle
6–Spine of scapula
7–Infraspinatus muscle
8–Superior lobe of left lung
9–Anastomosis of brachiocephalic
   veins with superior vena cava
10–Azygos vein
11–Left pulmonary artery
12–Inferior angle of left scapula
13–Left main bronchus
14–Left pulmonary artery
15–Lower esophagus
16–Inferior lobe of left lung
17–Spleen
18–Left suprarenal gland
19–Left colic flexure
20–Left kidney
21–Descending colon
22–Jejunum
23–Ala of ilium
24–Iliopsoas muscle
25–Femoral nerve
26–External iliac artery
27–External iliac vein
28–Gluteus minimus muscle
29–Gluteus medius muscle
30–Acetabulum
31–Head of left femur
32–Neck of left femur
33–Lesser trochanter
34–Left gluteus maximus muscle
35–Left semitendinosus muscle
36–Sciatic nerve
37–Left adductor magnus muscle
38–Obturator externus muscle
39–Clitoris
40–Left pubis
41–Right semitendinosus muscle
42–Right gluteus maximus muscle
43–Right adductor magnus muscle
44–Ossified upper shaft of right femur
45–Vastus lateralis muscle
46–Pubic symphysis
47–Neck of urinary bladder
48–Rectus femoris muscle
49–Left and right umbilical arteries
50–Ileum
51–Transversus abdominis muscle
52–Internal oblique abdominal muscle
53–External oblique abdominal
   muscle

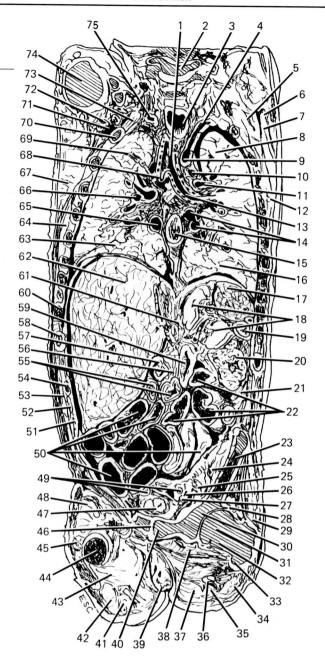

54–Right 10th costal cartilage
55–Inferior or horizontal part of
   duodenum
56–Head of pancreas
57–Descending part of duodenum
58–Right 9th costal cartilage
59–Duodenojejunal flexure
60–Right 8th rib
61–Supracrural part of diaphragm
62–Right lobe of liver
63–Inferior lobe of right lung
64–Serratus anterior muscle
65–Right pulmonary vein

66–Right pulmonary artery
67–Latissimus dorsi muscle
68–Right main bronchus
69–Superior lobe of right lung
70–Right 1st rib
71–Axillary vein
72–Axillary artery
73–Anterior scalene muscle
74–Head of right humerus
75–Subclavian artery
76–Stomach
77–Urinary bladder
78–Rib

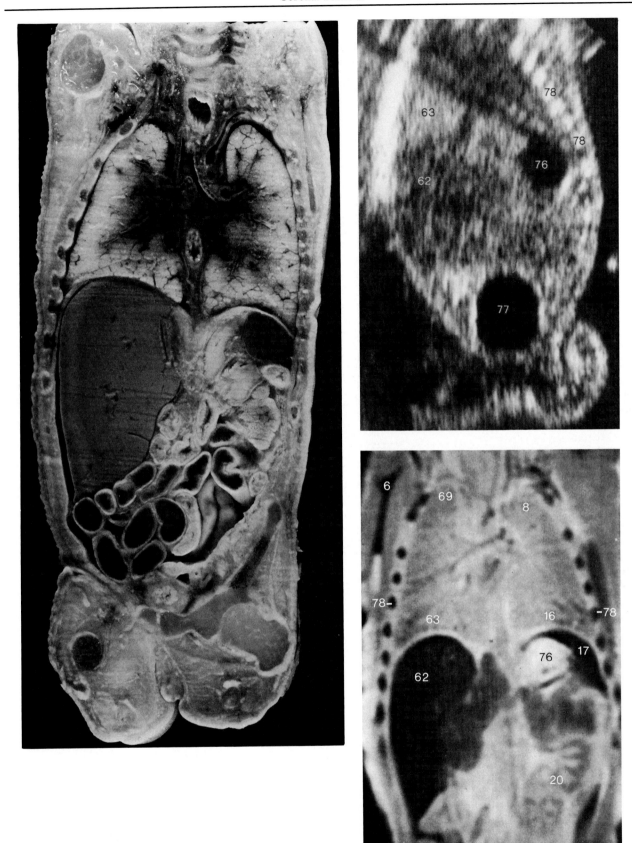

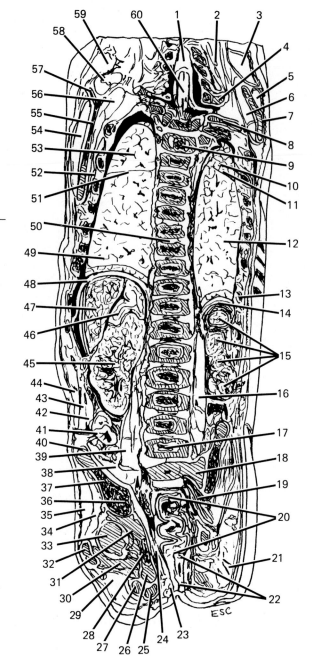

1–Dura mater
2–Multifidi muscles
3–Left trapezius muscle
4–Transverse process of C₇ vertebra
5–Left supraspinatus muscle
6–Left subscapularis muscle
7–Spine of left scapula
8–Left 1st rib
9–Ossification center of body of C₂
  vertebra
10–Superior lobe of left lung
11–Oblique fissure
12–Inferior lobe of left lung
13–Left 10th rib
14–Left side of diaphragm
15–Lobules of left kidney
16–Left psoas major muscle
17–Ossification center of body of L₅
  vertebra
18–Sacrum
19–S₁ spinal nerve
20–Rectum
21–Left gluteus maximus muscle
22–Anal canal
23–External anal sphincter muscle
24–Levator ani muscle
25–Origin of semitendinosus muscle
26–Tuberosity of ischium
27–Origin of long head of biceps
  femoris muscle
28–Ossification center of ischium
29–Right gluteus maximus muscle
30–Quadratus femoris muscle
31–Acetabulum
32–Greater trochanter
33–Head of right femur
34–Gluteus minimus muscle
35–Gluteus medius muscle
36–Body of ilium
37–Ala of ilium
38–Iliacus muscle
39–Right psoas major muscle
40–Crest of ilium
41–Ascending colon

42–Transversus abdominis muscle
43–Internal oblique abdominal muscle
44–External oblique abdominal
  muscle
45–Right kidney
46–Right suprarenal gland
47–Right lobe of liver
48–Right side of diaphragm

49–Inferior lobe of right lung
50–Intervertebral disc between T₇ and
  T₈ vertebrae
51–Oblique fissure
52–Serratus anterior muscle
53–Superior lobe of right lung
54–Infraspinatus muscle
55–Body of right scapula

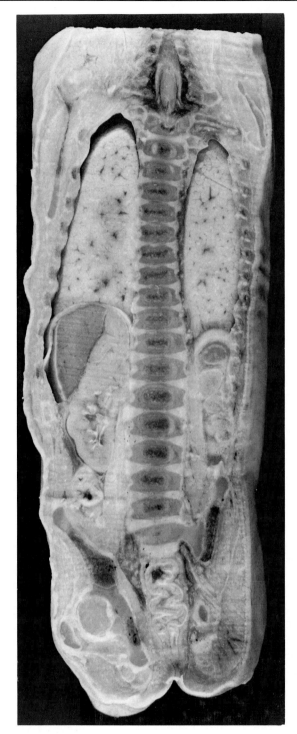

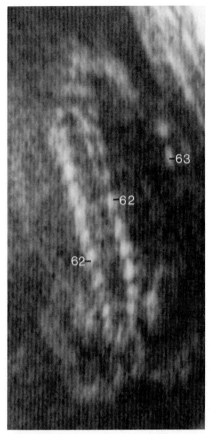

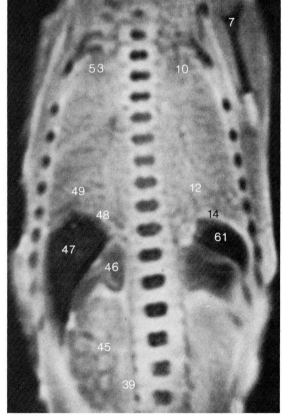

56–Right subscapularis muscle
57–Spine of right scapula
58–Right supraspinatus muscle
59–Right trapezius muscle
60–Spinal medulla (cord)
61–Spleen
62–Ossification center of lamina
63–Rib

Fetal Limbs

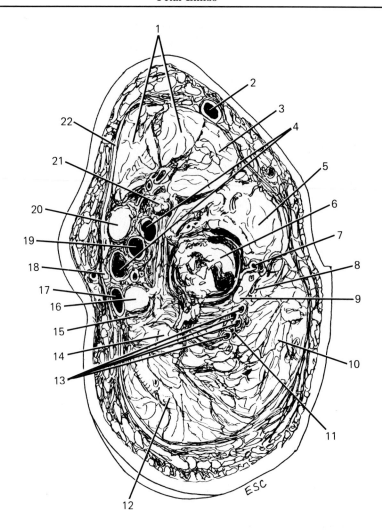

1–Biceps brachii muscle (short head)
2–Cephalic vein
3–Biceps brachii muscle (long head)
4–Brachial veins (venae comitantes of brachial artery)
5–Brachialis muscle
6–Midshaft of humerus
7–Radial collateral artery
8–Posterior antebrachial cutaneous nerve
9–Radial nerve
10–Triceps brachii muscle (lateral head)
11–Medial collateral artery
12–Triceps brachii muscle (long head)
13–Venae comitantes of medial collateral artery
14–Triceps brachii muscle (medial head)
15–Medial brachial intermuscular septum
16–Ulnar nerve
17–Basilic vein
18–Medial antebrachial cutaneous nerve
19–Brachial artery
20–Median nerve
21–Musculocutaneous nerve
22–Brachial fascia

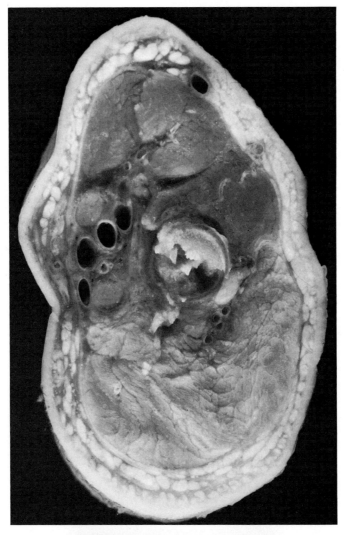

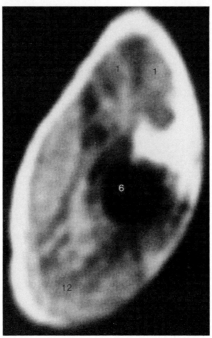

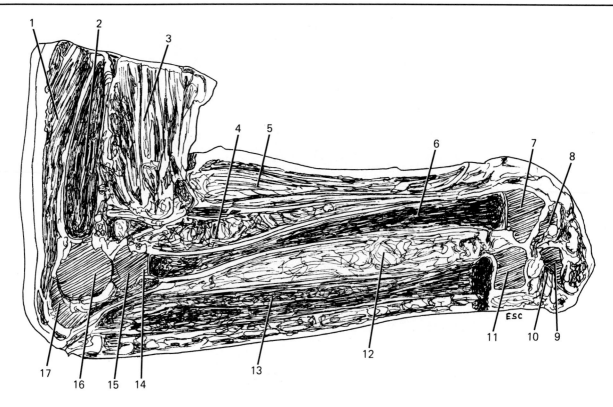

1–Triceps brachii muscle
2–Ossified shaft of humerus
3–Brachialis muscle
4–Pronator teres muscle
5–Brachioradialis muscle
6–Ossified shaft of radius
7–Distal epiphysis of radius
8–Carpal lunate cartilage (future bone)
9–Carpal triangular cartilage (future bone)
10–Articular disc
11–Distal epiphysis (head) of ulna
12–Antebrachial interosseous membrane
13–Ossified shaft of ulna
14–Neck of radius
15–Head of radius
16–Capitulum of humerus
17–Olecranon of ulna
18–Carpal cartilage
19–Phalangeal ossification center
20–Supraspinatus muscle
21–Infraspinatus muscle
22–Subscapularis muscle
23–Body of scapula
24–Rib

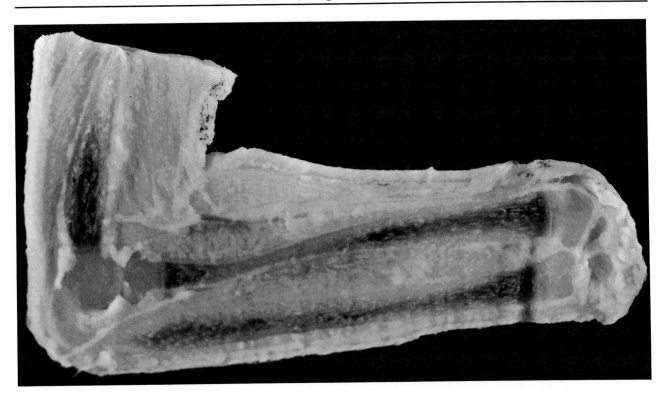

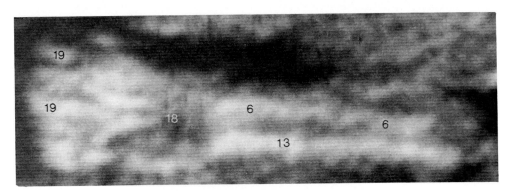

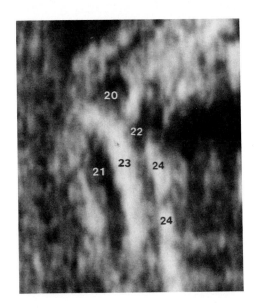

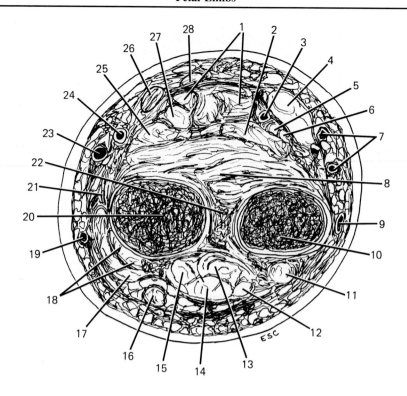

1–Flexor digitorum superficialis
  muscle
2–Flexor digitorum profundus
  muscle
3–Ulnar artery
4–Flexor carpi ulnaris muscle
5–Palmar branch of ulnar nerve
6–Dorsal branch of ulnar nerve
7–Median antebrachial veins
8–Pronator quadratus muscle
9–Basilic vein

10–Ulna
11–Extensor carpi ulnaris muscle
12–Extensor digiti minimi muscle
13–Extensor indicis muscle
14–Extensor digitorum muscle
15–Extensor pollicis longus muscle
16–Vein of dorsal venous plexus
17–Extensor pollicis brevis muscle
18–Tendons of extensor carpi radialis
  longus and brevis muscles
19–Vein of dorsal venous plexus

20–Radius
21–Tendon of brachioradialis muscle
22–Antebrachial interosseous
  membrane
23–Cephalic vein
24–Radial artery
25–Flexor pollicis longus muscle
26–Tendon of flexor carpi radialis
  muscle
27–Median nerve
28–Tendon of palmaris longus muscle

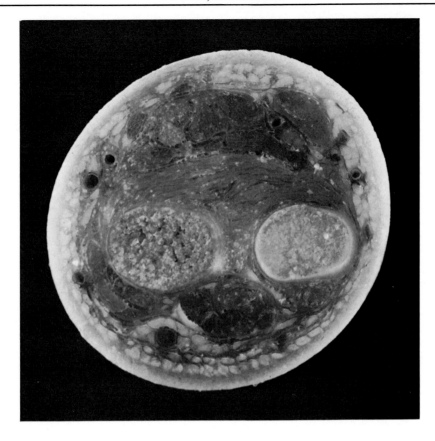

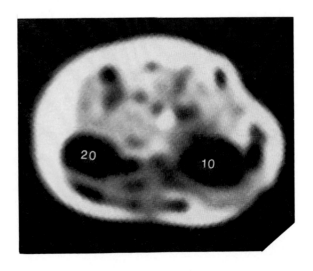

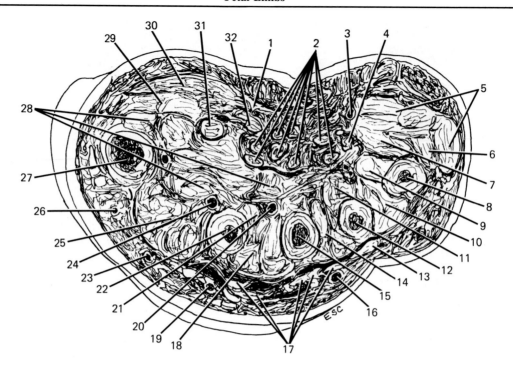

1–Palmar aponeurosis
2–Tendons of flexor digitorum
superficialis and profundus
muscles with accompanying
lumbrical muscles
3–Ulnar artery
4–Palmar branch of ulnar nerve
5–Abductor digiti brevis muscle
6–Flexor digiti minimi brevis muscle
7–Opponens digiti minimi muscle
8–5th metacarpal bone
9–3rd palmar interosseus muscle
10–4th dorsal interosseus muscle
11–2nd palmar interosseous muscle
12–4th metacarpal bone

13–Tendon of extensor digiti minimi
muscle
14–3rd dorsal interosseous muscle
15–3rd metacarpal bone
16–Vein of dorsal venous plexus
17–Tendons of extensor digitorum
muscle
18–2nd dorsal interosseous muscle
19–Vein of dorsal venous plexus
20–Deep palmar arterial arch
21–1st palmar interosseous muscle
22–2nd metacarpal bone
23–Vein of dorsal venous plexus
24–1st palmer metacarpal artery
25–1st dorsal interosseous muscle

26–Vein of dorsal venous plexus
27–1st metacarpal bone
28–Adductor pollicis muscle
29–Opponens pollicis muscle
30–Abductor pollicis brevis muscle
31–Tendon of flexor pollicis longus
muscle
32–Median nerve
33–Carpal cartilage
34–Metacarpal ossification center
35–Phalangeal ossification center
36–Ulna
37–Radius

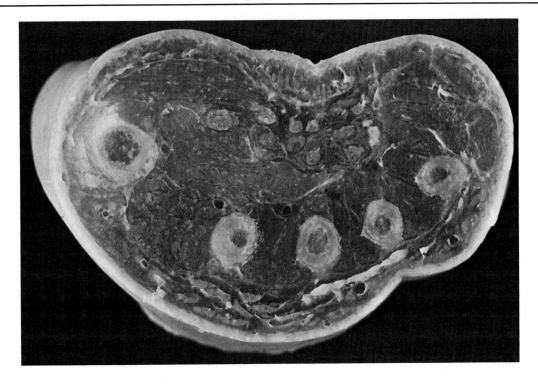

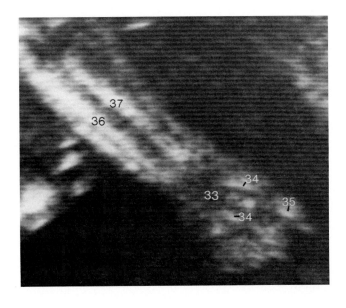

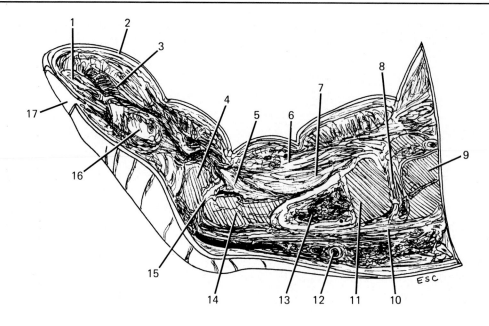

1–Tuberosity of head of distal
    phalanx
2–Epidermis
3–Dermis
4–Base of middle phalanx
5–One half of divided tendon of
    flexor digitorum superficialis
    muscle
6–Fibrous digital sheath
7–Tendon of flexor digitorum
    profundus muscle

8–Metacarpophalangeal joint
9–Head of 2nd metacarpal bone
10–Tendon of extensor digitorum
    muscle
11–Base of proximal phalanx of 2nd
    digit (index finger)
12–Branch of a dorsal digital vein
13–Ossified body of proximal phalanx
14–Head of proximal phalanx
15–Proximal interphalangeal joint

16–Articular capsule of distal
    interphalangeal joint
17–Nail
18–Distal cartilagenous end of radius
19–Radius
20–First metacarpal ossification
    center
21–Third metacarpal ossification
    center

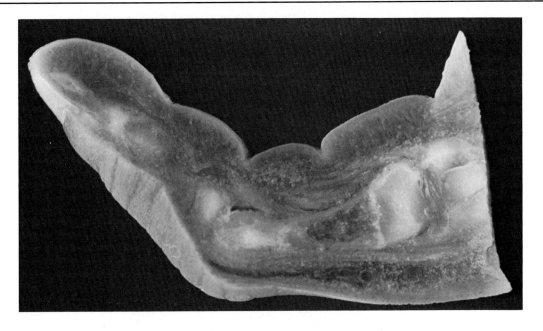

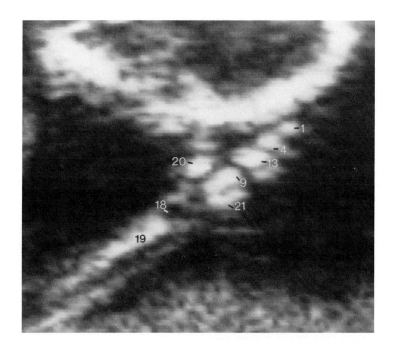

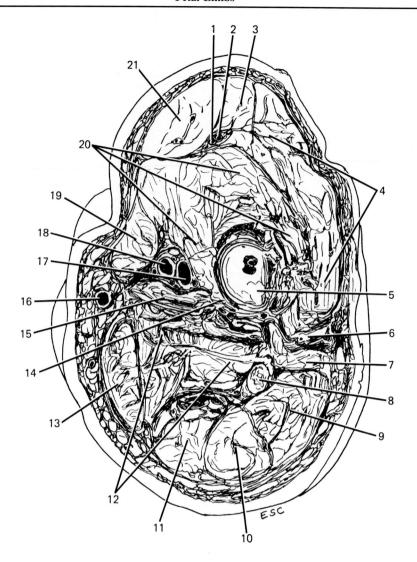

1–Femoral vein (in adductor canal)
2–Femoral artery (in adductor canal)
3–Rectus femoris muscle
4–Vastus lateralis muscle
5–Upper midshaft of femur
6–Lateral femoral intermuscular
   system
7–Gluteus maximus muscle

8–Sciatic nerve
9–Biceps femoris muscle (long head)
10–Semitendinosus muscle
11–Semimembranosus muscle
12–Adductor magnus muscle
13–Gracilis muscle
14–Medial femoral intermuscular
   septum

15–Adductor brevis muscle
16–Greater saphenous vein
17–Deep (profunda) femoral vein
18–Deep (profunda) femoral artery
19–Adductor longus muscle
20–Vasti intermedius and medialis
   muscles
21–Sartorius muscle

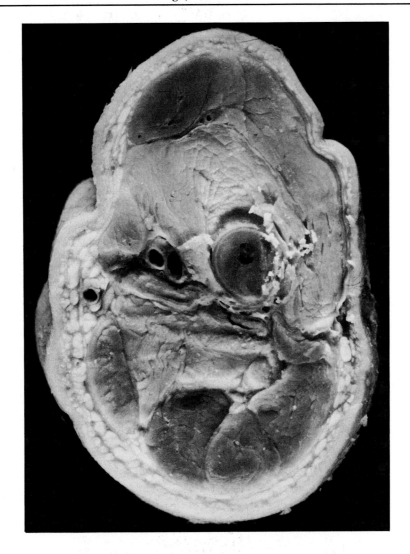

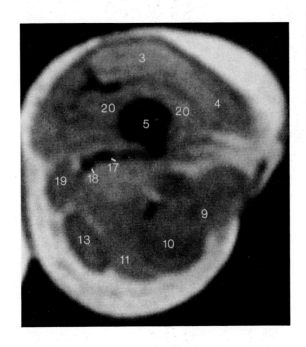

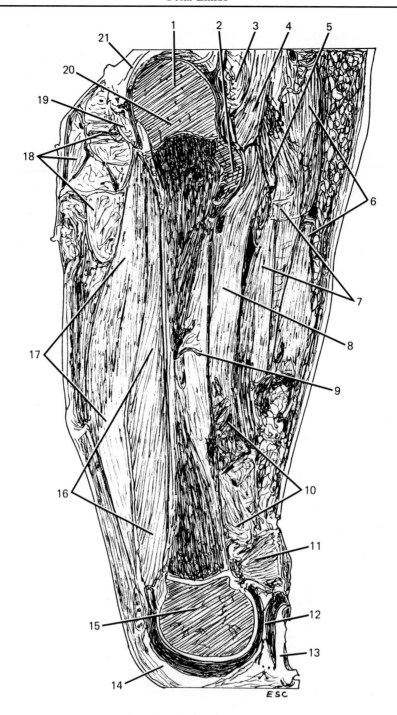

ESC

1–Head of femur
2–Lesser trochanter
3–Inferior gemellus muscle
4–Quadratus femoris muscle
5–Sciatic nerve
6–Semitendinosus muscle
7–Long head of biceps femoris
  muscle
8–Adductor magnus muscle
9–Nutrient arterial canal in midshaft
  of femur

10–Short head of biceps femoris
  muscle
11–Lateral head of gastrocnemius
  muscle
12–Lateral meniscus of flexed knee
  joint
13–Articular cartilage of lateral
  condyle of tibia
14–Capsule of knee joint
15–Lateral condyle of femur
16–Vastus intermedius muscle

17–Rectus femoris muscle
18–Sartorius muscle
19–Orbicular zone of hip joint capsule
20–Neck of femur
21–Acetabulum
22–Femoral diaphysis
23–Distal femoral epiphyseal
  ossification center—33 week
  gestation
24–Distal femoral epiphyseal cartilage
25–Fascial plane

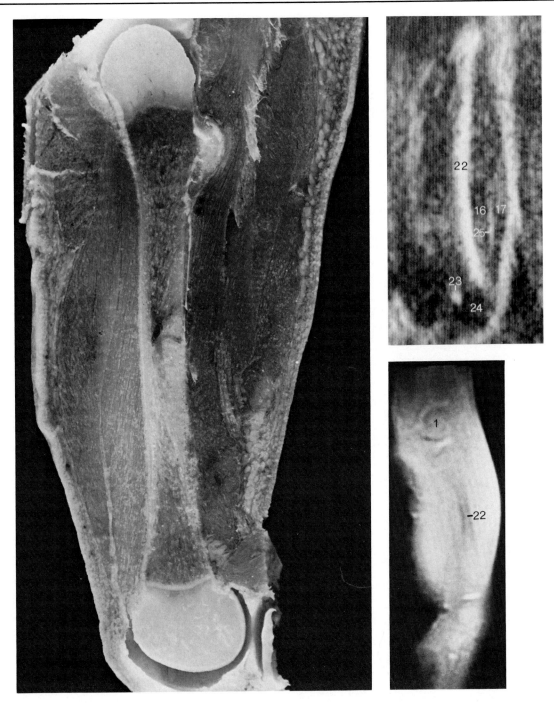

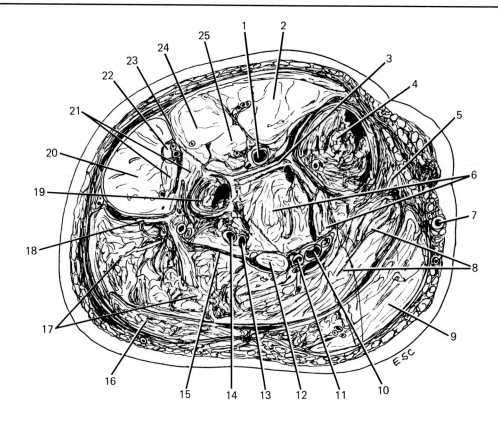

1–Anterior tibial artery
2–Tibialis anterior muscle
3–Crural interosseous membrane
4–Midshaft of tibia
5–Flexor digitorum longus muscle
6–Tibialis posterior muscle
7–Greater saphenous vein
8–Medial extent of soleus muscle
9–Medial head of gastrocnemius
  muscle
10–Posterior tibial artery

11–Posterior tibial vein
12–Tibial nerve
13–Fibular (peroneal) vein
14–Fibular (peroneal) artery
15–Transverse intermuscular septum
16–Lateral head of gastrocnemius
  muscle
17–Lateral extent of soleus muscle
18–Posterior crural intermuscular
  septum

19–Midshaft of fibula
20–Peroneus (fibularis) longus muscle
21–Peroneus (fibularis) brevis muscle
22–Superficial fibular (peroneal) nerve
23–Anterior crural intermuscular
  septum
24–Extensor digitorum longus muscle
25–Extensor hallucis longus muscle

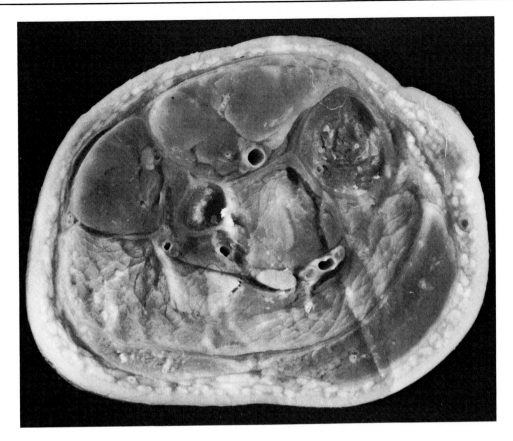

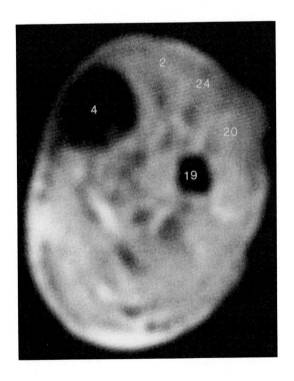

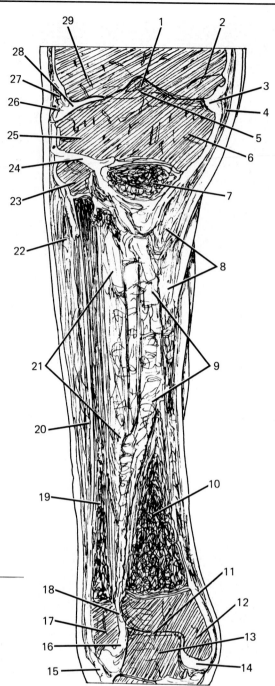

ESC

1–Anterior cruciate ligament
2–Medial condyle of femur
3–Medial meniscus of knee joint
4–Tibial collateral ligament
5–Intercondylar eminence of tibia
6–Medial condyle of tibia
7–Ossified proximal shaft of tibia
8–Soleus muscle
9–Periosteum lining posterior surface
  of shaft of tibia
10–Distal tibia
11–Talotibial part of ankle joint
12–Medial malleolus of tibia
13–Talus
14–Tibiotalar part of medial (deltoid)
   ligament
15–Calcaneofibular ligament
16–Talofibular part of ankle joint
17–Lateral malleolus of fibula
18–Tibiofibular joint

19–Ossified shaft of fibula
20–Peroneus (fibularis) longus muscle
21–Crural interosseous membrane
22–Peroneus (fibularis) brevis muscle
23–Head of fibula
24–Tibiofibular syndesmosis
25–Lateral condyle of tibia
26–Fibular collateral ligament
27–Tendon of origin of popliteus
   muscle
28–Lateral meniscus of knee joint

29–Lateral condyle of femur
30–Knee
31–Ankle
32–Dorsum of foot
33–Femur
34–Distal femoral ossification center
35–Proximal tibial ossification
   center—35 week gestation
36–Proximal tibia
37–Distal femoral epiphyseal cartilage
38–Proximal tibial epiphyseal cartilage

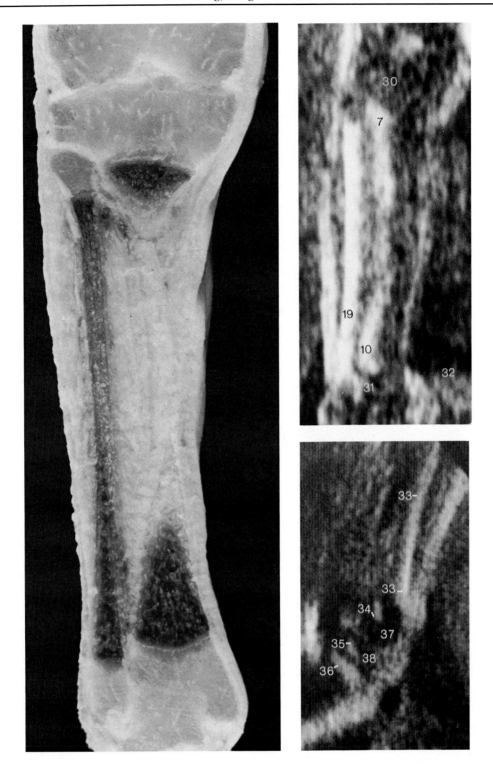

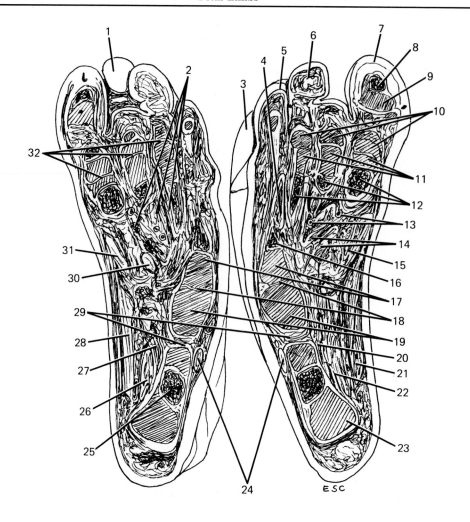

1–2nd digit
2–1st, 2nd and 3rd dorsal interosseous muscles
3–5th digit (minimus) (little toe)
4–2nd plantar interosseous muscle
5–4th digit
6–3rd digit
7–1st digit (hallux) (big toe)
8–Ossification center of body of distal phalanx
9–Base of distal phalanx
10–Base of proximal phalanges of 1st, 2nd and 3rd digits
11–Head of 1st, 2nd and 3rd metatarsal bones
12–Ossification center of body of 1st, 2nd and 3rd metatarsal bones
13–Common digital arteries
14–Oblique head of adductor hallucis muscle

15–Medial head of flexor hallucis brevis
16–Ossification center of body of 5th metatarsal bone
17–Base of 5th metatarsal bone
18–Cuboideometatarsal joint
19–Cuboid bone
20–Calcaneonavicular (spring) ligament
21–Abductor hallucis muscle
22–Quadratus plantae (accessory flexor) muscle
23–Tuberosity of calcaneus
24–Tendon of peroneus (fibularis) longus muscle
25–Ossification center of calcaneus
26–Quadratus plantae (accessory flexor) muscle
27–Calcaneonavicular (spring) ligament

28–Abductor hallucis muscle
29–Calcaneocuboid joint
30–Tendon (insertion) of peroneus (fibularis) muscle
31–Medial head of flexor hallucis brevis muscle
32–1st, 2nd and 3rd metatarsophalangeal joints
33–Distal metatarsal epiphyseal cartilage
34–Primary ossification center of metatarsal
35–Primary ossification center of calcaneus
36–Cartilagenous portion of calcaneus
37–Primary ossification center of talus

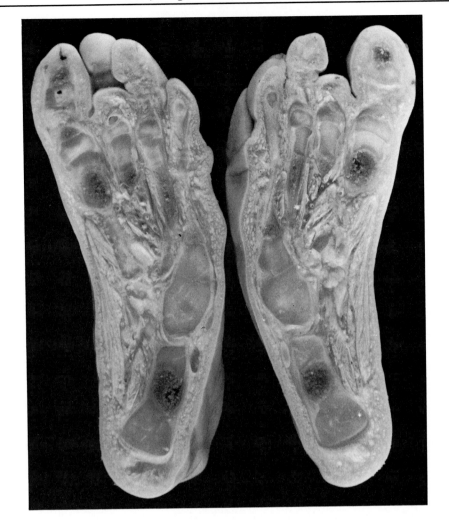

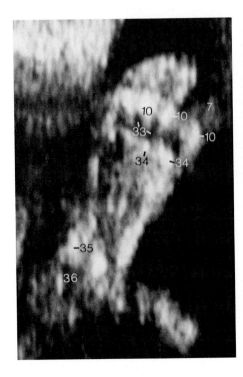

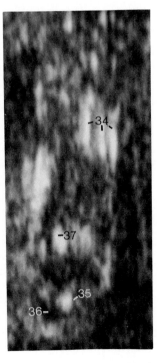

Special Studies

SECTION 1

Fetal Brain Development

Cortical Development
Ventricular Development
Dural Structures

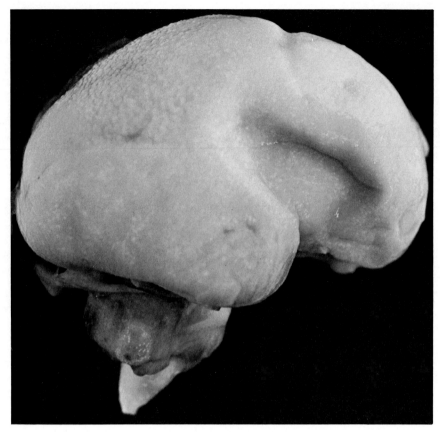

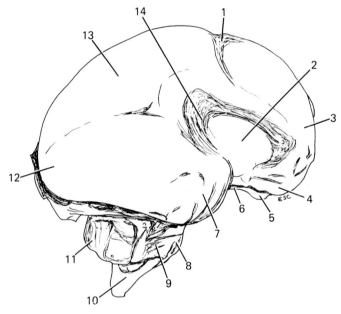

1–Central sulcus (of Rolando)
2–Insula (surface overlies corpus striatum [basal nuclei or ganglia])
3–Frontal lobe of right cerebral hemisphere
4–Lateral orbital gyrus

5–Olfactory bulb
6–Olfactory tract
7–Temporal lobe
8–Pons
9–Middle cerebral peduncle

10–Medulla oblongata
11–Right cerebellar hemisphere
12–Occipital lobe
13–Parietal lobe
14–Lateral sulcus (Sylvian fissure)

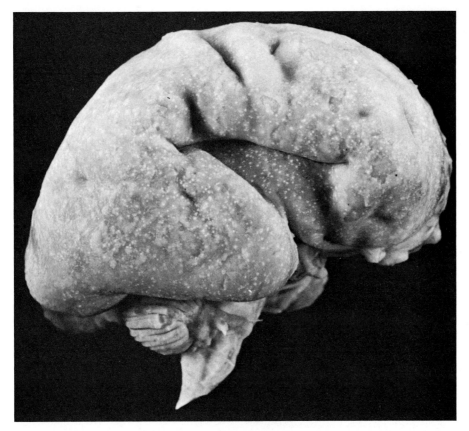

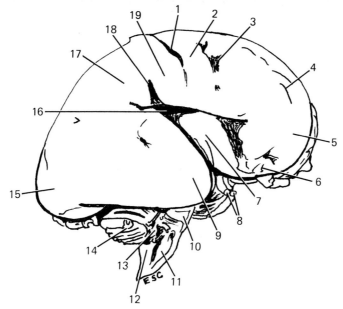

1–Central sulcus (of Rolando)
2–Precentral gyrus
3–Precentral sulcus
4–Superior frontal sulcus
5–Frontal lobe
6–Lateral orbital gyrus
7–Insula

8–Optic nerves
9–Temporal lobe
10–Pons
11–Olive
12–Medulla oblongata
13–Flocculus
14–Right cerebellar hemisphere

15–Occipital lobe
16–Lateral sulcus (of Sylvius)
17–Parietal lobe
18–Postcentral sulcus
19–Postcentral gyrus

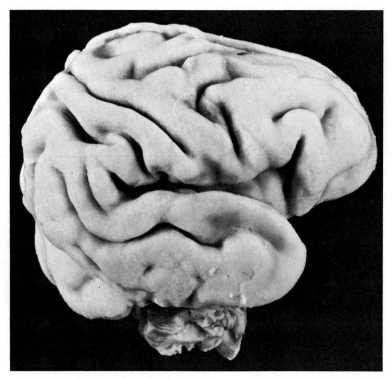

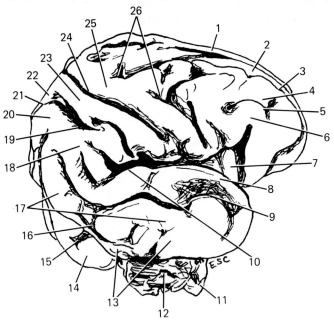

1–Superior frontal gyrus of left
  cerebral hemisphere
2–Superior frontal gyrus of right
  cerebral hemisphere
3–Superior frontal sulcus
4–Middle frontal gyrus
5–Inferior frontal sulcus
6–Inferior frontal gyrus
7–Insula
8–Superior temporal gyrus

9–Superior temporal sulcus
10–Lateral sulcus (of Sylvius)
11–Medulla oblongata
12–Right cerebellar hemisphere
13–Inferior temporal gyrus
14–Occipital lobe
15–Lateral occipital sulcus
16–Inferior temporal sulcus
17–Middle temporal gyrus

18–Supramarginal gyrus
19–Postcentral sulcus
20–Inferior parietal lobule
21–Interparietal sulcus
22–Superior parietal lobule
23–Postcentral gyrus
24–Central sulcus (of Rolando)
25–Precentral gyrus
26–Precentral sulcus

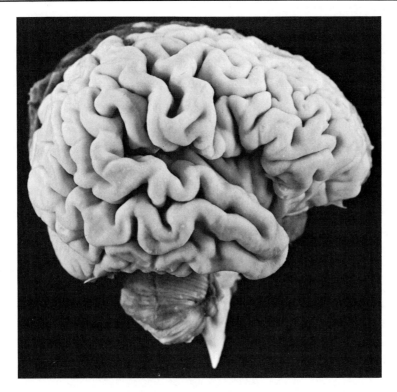

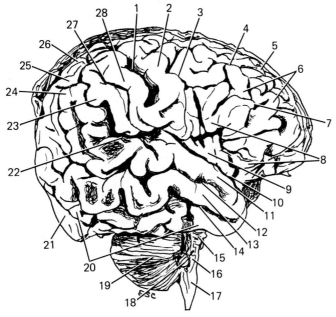

1–Central sulcus (of Rolando)
2–Precentral gyrus
3–Precentral sulcus
4–Superior frontal sulcus
5–Superior frontal gyrus
6–Middle frontal gyrus
7–Inferior frontal sulcus
8–Inferior temporal gyrus
9–Insula
10–Lateral sulcus (of Sylvius)

11–Superior temporal gyrus
12–Superior temporal sulcus
13–Middle temporal gyrus
14–Inferior temporal sulcus
15–Pons
16–Olive
17–Medulla oblongata
18–Flocculus
19–Right cerebellar hemisphere
20–Inferior temporal gyrus

21–Occipital lobe
22–Posterior ramus of lateral sulcus
   (of Sylvius)
23–Supramarginal gyrus
24–Angular gyrus
25–Inferior parietal lobule
26–Superior parietal lobule
27–Postcentral sulcus
28–Postcentral gyrus

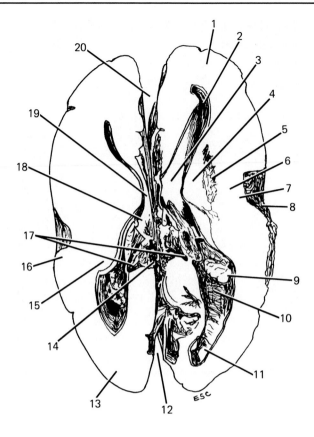

1–Frontal lobe
2–Anterior horn of left lateral
    ventricle
3–Body of lateral ventricle
4–Head of caudate nucleus
5–Internal capsule
6–Corpus striatum (basal nuclei or
    ganglia)
7–Insula

8–Lateral sulcus (of Sylvius)
9–Choroid plexus
10–Atrium of lateral ventricle
11–Posterior horn of lateral ventricle
12–Longitudinal cerebral fissure
13–Occipital lobe
14–Splenium of corpus callosum
15–Thalamus
16–Temporal lobe

17–Internal cerebral veins
18–Body of fornix
19–Lamina of septum pellucidum
20–Longitudinal cerebral fissure
21–Region of lateral wall of lateral
    ventricle
22–Medial wall of lateral ventricle
23–Falx/Interhemispheric fissure

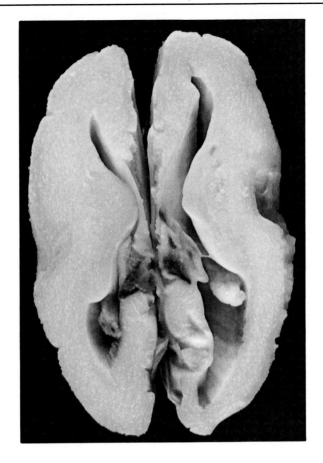

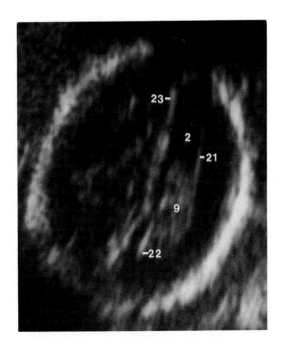

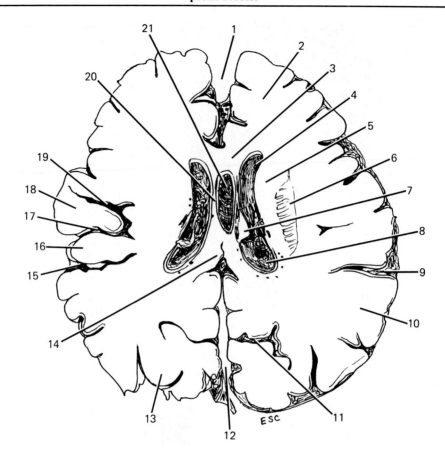

1–Longitudinal cerebral fissure
2–Frontal lobe
3–Genu of corpus callosum
4–Anterior horn of left lateral
   ventricle
5–Head of caudate nucleus
6–Internal capsule
7–Body of fornix
8–Atrium of lateral ventricle

9–Posterior ramus of lateral sulcus
   (of Sylvius)
10–Parietal lobe
11–Parieto-occipital sulcus
12–Longitudinal cerebral fissure
13–Occipital lobe
14–Splenium of corpus callosum
15–Posterior ramus of lateral sulcus
   (of Sylvius)

16–Postcentral gyrus
17–Central sulcus (of Rolando)
18–Precentral gyrus
19–Precentral sulcus
20–Lamina of septum pellucidum
21–Cavum of septum pellucidum
22–Falx/Interhemispheric fissure

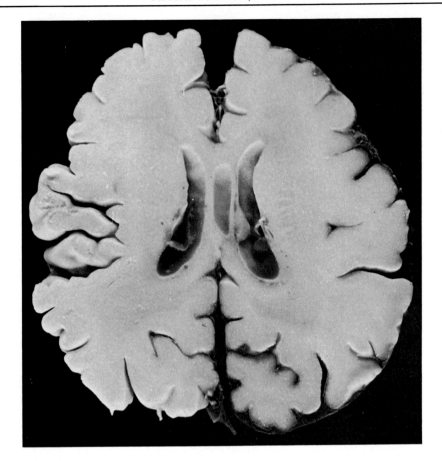

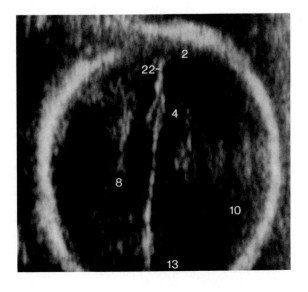

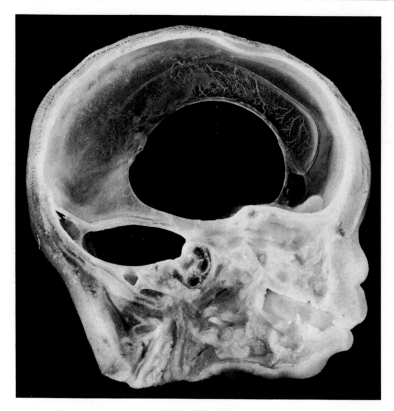

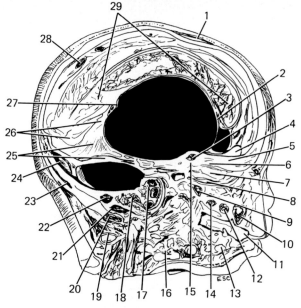

1–Anterior fonticulus (fontanelle)
2–Inferior sagittal sinus
3–Lesser wing of sphenoid
4–Crista galli
5–Roof of orbit (frontal bone)
6–Superior oblique muscle
7–Medial rectus muscle
8–Inferior rectus muscle
9–Greater wing of sphenoid bone
10–Upper deciduous canine tooth

11–Tongue
12–1st upper deciduous molar tooth
13–Mandible
14–2nd upper deciduous molar tooth
15–Superior orbital fissure
16–Submandibular gland
17–Cochlea
18–Petrous part of temporal bone
19–Posterior arch of atlas
20–Lateral part of occipital bone

21–Jugular bulb
22–Sigmoid sinus
23–Squamous part of occipital bone
24–Transverse sinus
25–Tentorium cerebelli
26–Location of straight sinus
27–Site where great cerebral vein
     joins straight sinus
28–Superior sagittal sinus
29–Falx cerebri

Special Studies

SECTION 2
Anatomy of the Ductus Venosus

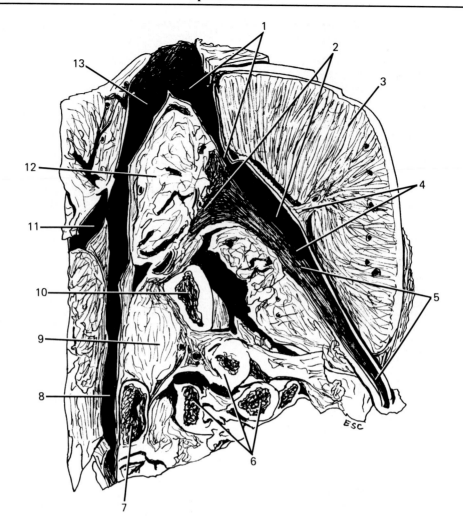

1–Ductus venosus
2–Left branch of portal vein
3–Left lobe of liver
4–Branches of left branch of portal
   vein
5–Umbilical vein

6–Jejunum
7–Inferior or horizontal part of
   duodenum
8–Inferior vena cava
9–Head of pancreas
10–Superior part of duodenum

11–Right suprarenal vein
12–Caudate lobe of liver
13–Inferior vena cava
14–Diaphragm

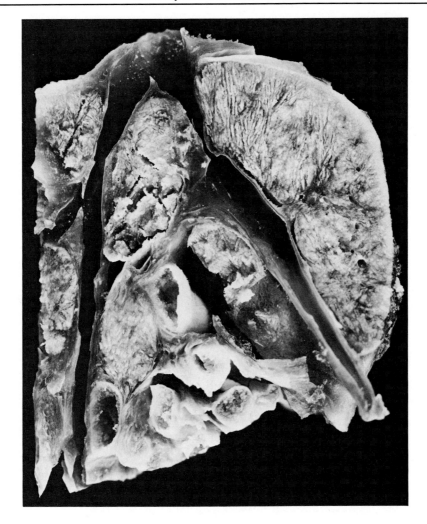

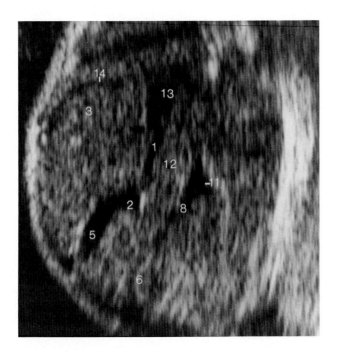

Special Studies

SECTION 3
Fetal Heart

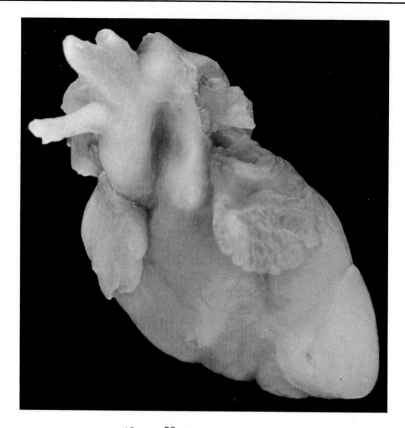

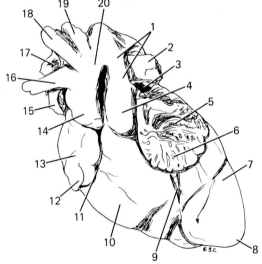

1–Ductus arteriosus
2–Left pulmonary artery
3–Left pulmonary vein
4–Pulmonary trunk
5–Left atrium
6–Auricle or atrial appendage of left atrium
7–Left ventricle

8–Apex
9–Anterior interventricular sulcus
10–Right ventricle
11–Coronary or atrioventricular sulcus
12–Auricle or atrial appendage of right atrium
13–Right atrium

14–Ascending aorta
15–Right pulmonary artery
16–Brachiocephalic artery
17–Superior vena cava
18–Left common carotid artery
19–Left subclavian artery
20–Arch of aorta

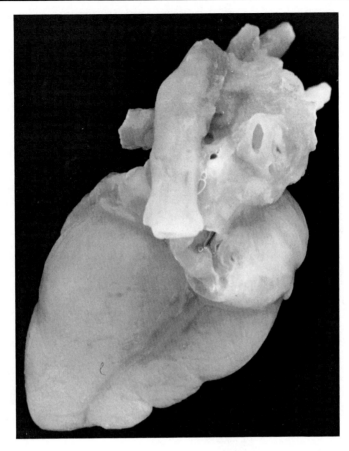

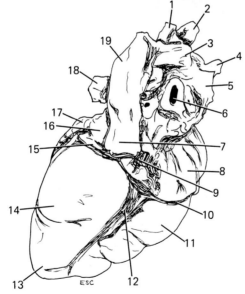

1–Left subclavian artery
2–Left common carotid artery
3–Superior vena cava
4–Brachiocephalic artery
5–Right pulmonary artery
6–Right pulmonary vein
7–Descending thoracic aorta
8–Right atrium

9–Inferior vena cava
10–Coronary or atrioventricular
sulcus
11–Right ventricle
12–Middle cardiac vein and posterior
interventricular branch of right
coronary artery in posterior
interventricular sulcus

13–Apex
14–Left ventricle
15–Circumflex branch of left coronary
artery
16–Coronary sinus
17–Left atrium
18–Left pulmonary artery
19–Arch of aorta

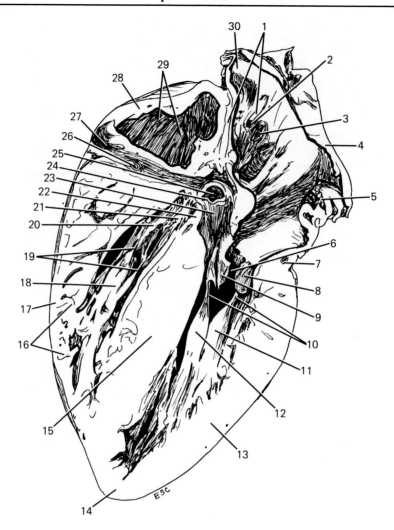

1–Interatrial septum
2–Upper anteriormost part of
   foramen ovale
3–Valve (septum primum) of
   foramen ovale
4–Left atrium
5–Left pulmonary vein
6–Left atrioventricular opening
7–Circumflex branch of left coronary
   artery
8–Posterior cusp of left
   atrioventricular (mitral) valve
9–Anterior cusp of left
   atrioventricular (mitral) valve
10–Chordae tendineae
11–Posterior papillary muscle

12–Anterior papillary muscle
13–Left ventricle
14–Apex
15–Muscular part of interventricular
    septum
16–Trabeculae carneae
17–Right ventricle
18–Anterior papillary muscle
19–Chordae tendineae
20–Anterior cusp of right
    atrioventricular (tricuspid) valve
21–Septal cusp of right
    atrioventricular (tricuspid) valve
22–Membranous part of
    interventricular septum

23–Lumen of origin of ascending
    aorta
24–Posterior valvula or aortic
    semilunar valve
25–Aortic sinus
26–Right coronary artery in coronary
    sulcus
27–Small cardiac vein
28–Right atrium
29–Musculi pectinati
30–Right pulmonary vein
31–Descending aorta
32–Spine
33–Aortic root

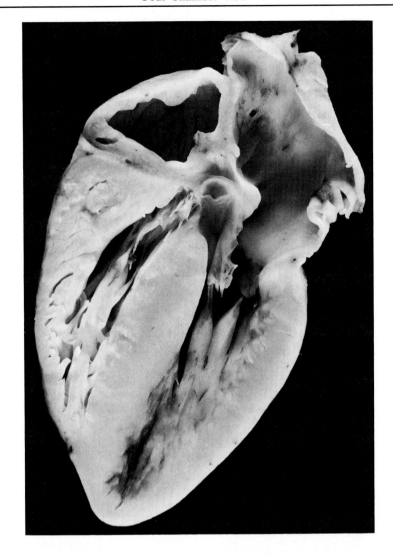

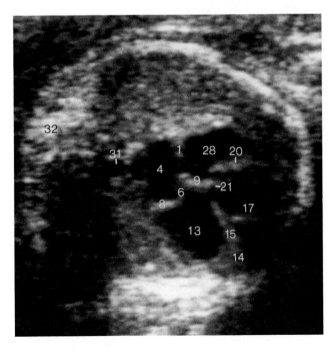

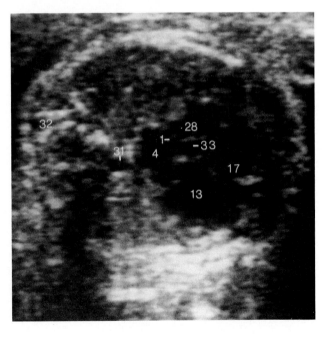

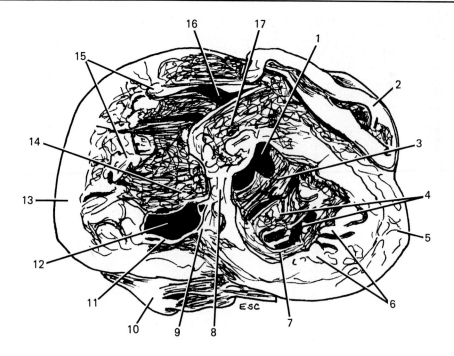

1–Opening into ascending aorta
2–Auricle or atrial appendage of the
  left atrium
3–Anterior cusp of left
  atrioventricular (mitral) valve
4–Chordae tendineae
5–Left ventricle
6–Trabeculae carneae
7–Posterior cusp of left
  atrioventricular (mitral) valve

8–Interventricular septum
  (membranous part)
9–Septal cusp of right
  atrioventricular (tricuspid) valve
10–Coronary sinus
11–Posterior cusp of right
  atrioventricular (tricuspid) valve
12–Right atrioventricular opening
13–Right ventricle

14–Anterior cusp of right
  atrioventricular (tricuspid) valve
15–Trabeculae carneae
16–Opening into pulmonary trunk
17–Interventricular septum (muscular
  part)

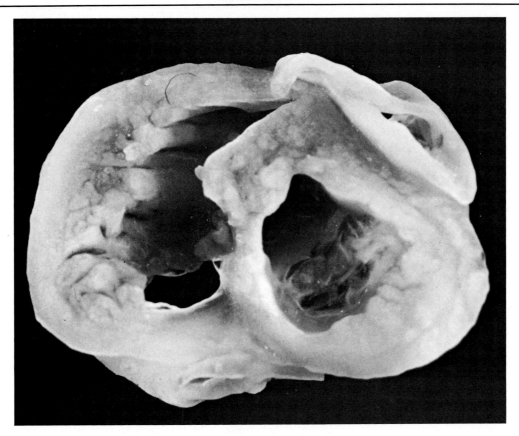

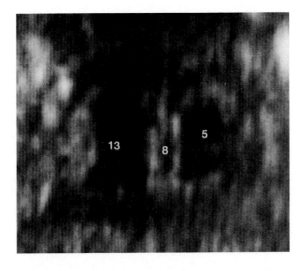

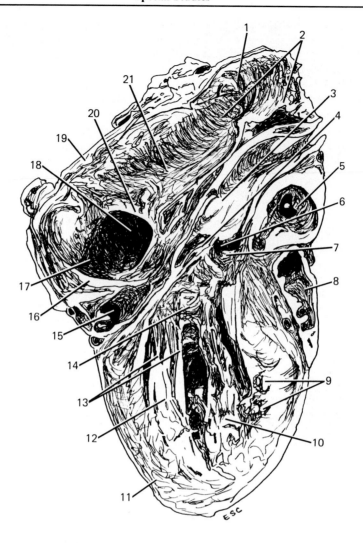

1–Opening of azygous vein
2–Superior vena cava
3–Ascending aorta
4–Posterior valvula or semilunar
  valve of aorta
5–Pulmonary trunk
6–Opening of left coronary artery
  into aortic sinus
7–Left valvula or semilunar valve of
  aorta
8–Auricle or atrial appendage of left
  atrium

9–Trabeculae carneae
10–Anterior papillary muscles
11–Left ventricle
12–Posterior papillary muscles
13–Chordae tendineae
14–Anterior cusp of left
  atrioventricular (mitral) valve
15–Opening of coronary sinus into
  right atrium
16–Valve of inferior vena cava
  (borders opening of inferior vena
  cava into right atrium)

17–Sinus venarum
18–Valve (septum primum) forming
  wall of fossa ovalis
19–Right atrium
20–Limbus of fossa ovalis
21–Interatrial septum
22–Left atrium
23–Right ventricle
24–Aortic valve

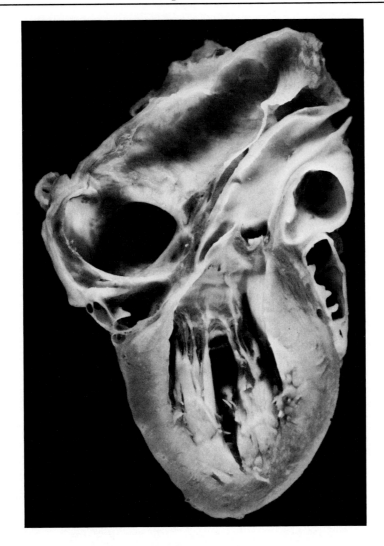

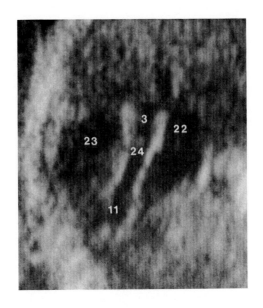

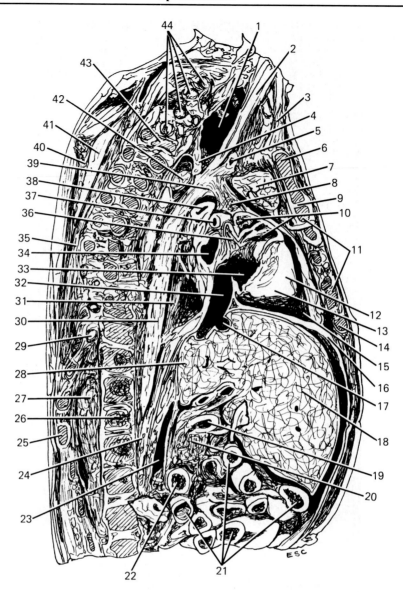

ESC

1–Prevertebral fascial cleft
(artifactually enlarged)
2–Left common carotid artery
3–Infrahyoid (strap) muscles
4–Left subclavian artery
5–Brachiocephalic artery
6–Manubrium of sternum
7–Thymus gland
8–Ascending aorta
9–Sternal angle
10–Auricle or atrial appendage of
right atrium
11–Cartilagenous sternebrae (future
body of sternum)
12–Left ventricle
13–Right ventricle
14–Xiphoid process
15–Pericardial cavity

16–Diaphragm
17–Ductus venosus
18–Left lobe of liver
19–Superior part of duodenum
20–Head of pancreas
21–Jejunum
22–Inferior or horizontal part of
duodenum
23–Inferior vena cava
24–Right crus of diaphragm
25–Spinous process of L_1 vertebra
26–Ossification center of body of L_1
vertebra
27–Left spinal nerve roots in vertebral
canal
28–Caudate lobe of liver
29–Sensory ganglion of left T_{10} spinal
nerve in intervertebral foramen

30–Descending thoracic aorta
31–Esophagus
32–Inferior vena cava
33–Right atrium
34–Right pulmonary vein joining left
atrium
35–Latissimus dorsi muscle
36–Superior vena cava
37–Right pulmonary artery
38–Right main bronchus
39–Arch of aorta
40–Trapezius muscle
41–Rhomboideus major muscle
42–Superior lobe of left lung
43–Body of T_2 vertebra
44–Left C_{5-8} spinal nerves
45–Spine

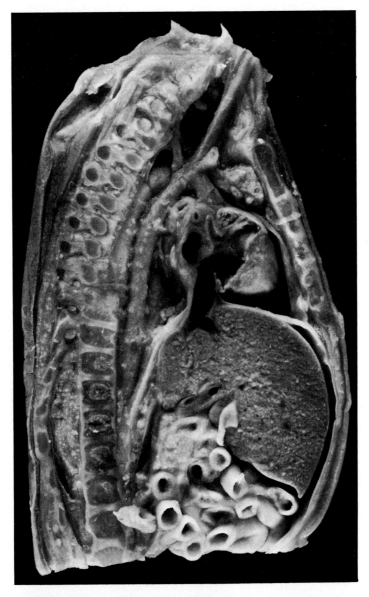

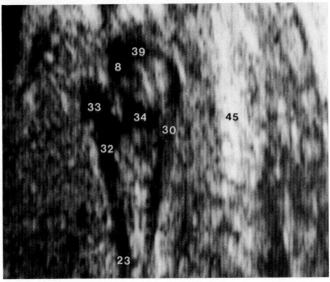

Index

Acetabulum
  axial section, 86, 87
  coronal section, 122–125
  longitudinal section, 140, 141
  sagittal section, 106, 107, 116, 117
Anal canal, 100, 101, 110, 111, 124, 125
Anal sphincter
  external
    axial section, 90, 91, 100, 101
    coronal section, 124, 125
    sagittal section, 110, 111
  internal, 90, 91, 100, 101
Ankle, 144, 145
Anus, 90, 91
Aorta
  arch of, 110, 111, 164, 165, 172, 173
  ascending, 164, 166-173
    axial section, 62, 63
    sagittal section, 110, 111
  axial section, 72–79
  descending, 165, 166, 172, 173
    axial section, 62, 63, 66–71
    sagittal section, 110, 111
  root of, 166
Aponeurosis, palmar, 134, 135
Appendix
  axial section, 78, 79
  sagittal section, 114, 115
Arteries
  axillary
    axial section, 60, 61
    coronal section, 122, 123
    sagittal section, 104, 105
  basilar, 4, 5, 42
  brachiocephalic, 164, 165, 172, 173
    axial section, 60, 61
    sagittal section, 112, 113
  carotid
    common, 52–55, 58–61, 164, 165, 172, 173
    external, 8, 9, 50, 51
    internal, 20, 21, 46, 47, 50, 51
  cerebellar, posterior-inferior, 28, 29
  cerebral
    anterior, 42
    middle, 16–19, 24, 25, 42
  cervical, transverse, 106, 107
  communicating, posterior, 22, 23
  coronary, 165-167, 170, 171
  digital, common, 146, 147
  femoral, 86, 87, 138, 139
  fibular (peroneal), 142, 143
  hepatic, proper, 72, 73
  iliac
    common, 80, 81, 110, 111

    external, 84, 85, 94, 95, 122, 123
    internal, 84, 85, 94, 95
  maxillary, 10, 11
  metacarpal, palmar, 134, 135
  occipital, 22, 23
  palatine, ascending, 20, 21
  palmar arch of, deep, 134, 135
  of penis, dorsal, 88, 89
  pudendal, internal, 88, 89
  pulmonary, 164, 165, 172, 173
    coronal section, 122, 123
    sagittal section, 108–113
  pulmonary trunk, 164, 168–171
    axial section 62, 63
    coronal section, 120, 145
    sagittal section, 110, 111
  radial, 132, 133
  rectal, superior, 80, 81
  subclavian, 164, 165, 172, 173
    axial section, 60, 61
    sagittal section, 106–109, 114, 115
  tibial
    anterior, 142, 143
    posterior, 142, 143
  ulnar, 132–135
  umbilical
    coronal section, 120–123
    sagittal section, 108–111
  vertebral, 52, 53, 58, 59
Atlas
  anterior arch of, 4, 5, 50, 51
  lateral mass of, 6, 7, 24, 25, 50, 51
  posterior arch of, 2–5, 26–29, 50, 51, 158
  transverse ligament of, 50, 51
Axis
  dens of, 4, 5, 24, 25, 50, 51
  ossification center of, 24, 25
  spinous process of, 2–5

Bile duct, common, 74, 75, 120, 121
Bladder, urinary
  axial section, 80, 84, 85, 94–97
  coronal section, 122, 123
  sagittal section, 108–111
Bones
  clavicle
    axial section, 58–61
    coronal section, 120, 145
    sagittal section, 104–109, 112–117
  coccyx
    axial section, 88–91, 100, 101
    sagittal section, 110, 111
  cranial. See Cranial bones
  facial. See Facial bones

  of foot, 146, 147
  of hand, 133-137
  of hip
    ilium. See Ilium
    ischium
      axial section, 86, 87, 96, 97
      coronal section, 124, 125
      sagittal section, 108, 109
    pubis. See Pubis
  hyoid
    axial section, 50, 51
    coronal section, 18–21
    sagittal section, 2–7
  of lower limb
    femur. See Femur
    fibula
      cross-section, 142, 143
      head of, 144, 145
      longitudinal section, 144, 145
      malleolus of, lateral, 144, 145
    tibia. See Tibia
  of upper limb
    humerus. See Humerus
    phalanx. See Phalanx
    radius. See Radius
    ulna. See Ulna
  mandible. See Mandible
  maxilla
    axial section, 46, 47
    coronal section, 14–17
    sagittal section, 4, 5
  ribs. See Ribs
  sacrum. See Sacrum
  scapula. See Scapula
  of skull. See Skull
  sternum. See Sternum
  vertebrae. See Vertebrae
Brain
  amygdala, 20, 21
  arachnoid membrane, 18–21, 24–30, 54, 55
  caudate nucleus, 154–157
    axial section, 38–41
    coronal section, 20–23
  cerebellar hemisphere, 150–153
    axial section, 42, 44, 45
    sagittal section, 2, 3, 6, 7
  cerebellar peduncle,
    middle, 24, 25, 26, 27, 42, 43
    superior, 2, 3, 26, 27
  cerebellar pyramis, 42, 43
  cerebellar tonsil, 42, 43
  cerebellomedullaris cistern
    axial section, 42–45
    coronal section, 26–29
    sagittal section, 4, 5

Brain (*cont.*)
  cerebellum, 150–153
    axial section, 40, 41
    coronal section, 26–29
    flocculus of, 44, 45, 151, 153
    sagittal section, 4, 5, 8, 9
    vermis of, 28, 29, 42
  cerebral aqueduct (of Sylvius), 40, 41
  cerebral hemisphere, 32, 33
  cerebral peduncle, 150
    axial section, 40–43
    coronal section, 24, 25
    sagittal section, 4, 5
  cerebrospinal fluid, 16, 17, 20, 22
  chiasmatic cistern, 2, 3, 42
  choroid plexus, 154, 155
    axial section, 38, 39
    coronal section, 26, 27
    sagittal section, 6-8
  cingulate gyrus, 2, 3, 36, 37
  cistern
    cerebellomedullaris, *See* cerebellome-
      dullaris cistern
    chiasmatic, 2, 3, 42
    interpeduncular, 22, 23, 42
    magna, 4, 5
    of great cerebral vein
      axial section, 38–40
      coronal section, 26, 27
      sagittal section, 4, 5
  cisterna magna, 4, 5
  colliculi
    inferior, 2–5, 26, 27, 40, 41
    superior, 2–5, 26, 27, 38, 39
  commissure
    anterior, 40, 41
    posterior, 38, 39
  corpus callosum
    axial section, 38, 39
    coronal section, 20–25
    genu of, 156, 157
    sagittal section, 2-5
    splenium of, 4, 5, 154–157
    sulci of, 2–5, 20, 21
  corpus striatum, 154, 155
    axial section, 38–41
    coronal section, 20–23
  dura mater
    axial section, 40, 41, 48–55
    coronal section, 14–21, 24, 25, 30
  falx cerebri, 154, 156, 158
    axial section, 32–41
    coronal section, 14–30
  fissures. (Also *see* Sulci)
    calcarine, 2, 3
    cerebral, lateral (Sylvian), 8–11, 20–
      25,38, 39
    cerebral, longitudinal, 20–25, 34, 35,
      154, 157
    choroid fissure, 2–5, 22–25, 40, 41
    falx/interhemispheric, 34, 35, 38, 39,
      154, 156
    orbital, superior, 158
    petro-occipital, 24, 25
  fornix, 154–157
    axial section, 38, 39
    coronal section, 22, 23
    sagittal section, 2, 3
  frontal lobe, 150, 151, 154–157
    axial section, 36–43
    coronal section, 14–19
    sagittal section, 2, 4–11

gyri
  angular, 153
  cingulate, 2, 3, 36, 37
  frontal
    inferior, 152
    middle, 152, 153
    superior, 152, 153
  orbital, 42, 43, 150, 151
  parahippocampal, 24, 25, 40, 41
  postcentral, 151–153, 156, 157
  precentral, 151–153, 156, 157
  straight, 42, 43
  supramarginal, 152, 153
  temporal
    inferior, 152, 153
    middle, 152, 153
    superior, 152, 153
hippocampus
  axial section, 38–41
  coronal section, 22–27
  sagittal section, 6–9
hypothalamus, 2, 3
infundibulum, 20, 21, 42, 43
insula, 150–155
  axial section, 38–41
  coronal section, 20–23
  sagittal section, 8, 9,
internal capsule, 22, 23, 38–41, 154–157
interpeduncular fossa, 40, 41
interthalamic adhesion, 38, 39
jugular bulb, 158
  axial section, 44, 45, 48, 49
  coronal section, 26–29
mamillary body, 22, 23, 42, 43
medulla oblongata, 150-153
  axial section, 42–47
  coronal section, 24–27
  sagittal section, 4, 5
midbrain, 2, 42
occipital lobe, 150–157
  axial section, 36–41
  coronal section, 28–30
  sagittal section, 2–11
olfactory area, 20, 21
olfactory bulb, 16, 17, 150
olfactory tract, 4, 5, 18, 19, 150
olive, 2–5, 151, 153
optic chiasma, 42, 43
optic tract, 20, 21
orbital gyri, 42, 43, 150, 151
parahippocampal gyrus, 24, 25, 40, 41
parietal lobe, 150–153, 156, 157
  axial section, 36, 37
  coronal section, 20–29
  sagittal section, 2–11
parietal lobule, superior, 32–35
pituitary gland, 2–5
pituitary stalk, 42, 43
pons, 150, 151, 153
  axial section, 42–45
  sagittal section, 2, 4, 5
postcentral gyrus, 32–35, 151–153, 156,
  157
precentral gyrus, 32–35, 151–153, 156, 157
    septum pellucidum
  axial section, 38, 39
  cavum of, 156
  coronal section, 18, 20, 21
  lamina of, 154, 155
  sagittal section, 4, 5
sinuses
  cavernous, 22, 23, 44, 45

confluence of, 4, 5, 30, 40, 41
  sagittal
    inferior, 158
    superior, 4, 5, 16–30, 32–41, 158
  sigmoid, 10, 11, 28, 29, 48, 49, 158
  straight, 2–5, 28–30, 38, 39, 158
  transverse, 2, 3, 6, 7, 10, 11, 28–30,
    42, 43, 158
straight gyrus, 42, 43
subarachnoid space, 24–30, 38–40, 54,
  55
subdural space, 16–25, 28–30
sulci
  calcarine, 4, 5, 28–30
  central (of Rolando), 8–11, 32–37,
    150–153, 156, 157
  cerebral, lateral (Sylvian), 8–11, 20–
    25, 38, 39
  corpus callosum, 2–5, 20–25
  frontal
    inferior, 14, 15, 152, 153
    superior, 151–153
  hippocampal, 22, 23
  interparietal, 152
  occipital, 152
  orbital, 42, 43
  parieto-occipital, 2–5, 36, 37, 156, 157
  postcentral, 151–153
  precentral, 151, 153, 156, 157
  temporal
    inferior, 152, 153
    superior, 152, 153
temporal gyri, 152, 153
temporal lobe, 150, 151, 154, 155
  axial section, 38–43
  coronal section, 18, 20, 21
  sagittal section, 6-11
  uncus of, 22, 33
tentoruium cerebelli, 158
  axial section, 40–43
  coronal section, 24–30
  sagittal section, 6–9,
thalamus, 154, 155
  axial section, 38–41
  coronal section, 22–27
  sagittal section, 2–7
tuber cinereum, 20, 21, 42, 43
ventricles. *See* Ventricles of brain
Bulb
  jugular, 158
    axial section, 44, 45, 48, 49
    coronal section, 26–29
  olfactory, 16, 17, 150

Calcaneus, 146, 147
Cartilage
  arytenoid, 2, 3
  carpal, 130, 134
    lunate, 130, 131
    triangular, 130, 131
  costal
    1st, 60, 61, 108, 109, 120, 121
    2nd, 62, 63, 106, 107
    3rd, 112, 113
    4th, 64, 65, 116, 117
    5th, 64–67, 104, 105, 116, 117
    6th, 66–69, 104, 105, 116, 117
    7th, 66–71, 106-113, 116, 117, 120, 121
    8th, 70, 71, 114–117
    9th, 122–125
    10th, 74, 75, 122, 123

cricoid
  axial section, 52–55
  sagittal section, 112, 113
ethmoid, 14, 15
nasal, lateral, 44–47
thyroid, 124, 145
  axial section, 50–55
  coronal section, 20, 21
  sagittal section, 6, 7
Cauda equina, 110, 111
  axial section, 80, 81, 84–87, 94–97
Choroid plexus, 154, 155
  axial section, 38, 39
  coronal section, 26, 27
  sagittal section, 6–8
Cistern
  cerebellomedullaris
    axial section, 42–45
    coronal section, 26–29
    sagittal section, 4, 5
  chiasmatic, 2, 3, 42
  chyli, 72, 73
  of great cerebral vein, 4, 5, 26, 27, 38–40
  interpeduncular, 22, 23, 42
  magna, 4, 5
Clavicle
  axial section, 58–61
  coronal section, 120, 145
  sagittal section, 104–109, 112–117
Coccyx
  axial section, 88–91, 100, 101
  sagittal section, 110, 111
Colliculus
  inferior, 2–5, 26, 27, 40, 41
  superior, 2–5, 26, 27, 38, 39
Colon
  ascending, 76–79, 124, 125
  colic flexure of, 122, 123
  descending, 74–81, 122, 123
  sigmoid, 110-113
  splenic flexure of, 104, 105
  transverse, 76–79, 106–113
Commissures
  of brain
    anterior, 40, 41
    posterior, 38, 39
  palpebral, lateral, 10, 11
Concha
  inferior
    coronal section, 14–17
    sagittal section, 4, 5
  middle, 14–17
  sphenoid, 18, 19
Costal cartilage. See Cartilage, costal
Cranial bones
  frontal
    axial section, 38–43
    coronal section, 14–19
    sagittal section, 2–11
  occipital. See Occipital bone
  parietal
    axial section, 32–35, 38–43
    coronal section, 20–24, 26, 28, 29
    sagittal section, 2–11
  sphenoid.See Sphenoid bone
  temporal. See Temporal bone
Cranial fossae
  anterior, 18, 19, 40, 41, 44, 45
  middle, 10, 11, 18, 19, 40–45
  posterior, 26, 27, 44, 45
Cranial nerves
  abducens, 20, 21, 44, 45

facial nerve, 44–49
oculomotor nerve, 2–5, 20–23, 42, 43
ophthalmic, 20, 21
optic, 2-5, 44, 45, 151
trochlear, 20, 21
vagus, 50–55, 58–61
Crista galli, 158
  coronal section, 14, 15
  sagittal section, 2, 3

Diaphragm, 68, 69, 160, 172, 173
  axial section, 66–77
  coronal section, 120–125
  sagittal section, 104–117
  urogenital
    axial section, 98, 99
    sagittal section, 110, 111
Digits
  of foot, 146, 147
  of hand, 136, 137
Dura mater
  of brain
    axial section, 40, 41, 48–55
    coronal section, 14–21, 24, 25, 30
  of cauda equina, 110, 111
  of spinal medulla, 58, 59, 110, 111, 124, 125

Ears
  acoustic meatus
    external, 22, 23, 46–49
  auditory tube of, 46–49
  auricle of, 20, 21, 24, 25, 44–47
  cochlea of, 158
    axial section, 44–47
    coronal section, 22, 23
    sagittal section, 6–9
  cochlear nerve of, 6, 7
  ear ridge, 24
  eardrum, 22, 23, 46, 47
  incus of, 10, 11
  inner, 24, 25
  malleus, 10, 11, 22, 23, 46, 47
  middle, 8, 9, 44, 45, 46, 47
  oval window of, 8, 9
  promontory, 8, 9
  round window of, 8, 9
  semicircular canal of
    anterior, 8, 9, 24, 25
    crus commune, 8
    lateral, 8, 9, 24, 25
    posterior, 24, 44–47
  stapedius muscle of, 46, 47
  tympanic cavity
    axial section, 44, 45, 48, 49
    coronal section, 22, 23
    sagittal section, 8–11
  tympanic membrane
    axial section, 46–49
    coronal section, 22, 23
  tympanic ring of, 48, 49
  vestibule of
    axial section, 44, 45, 48, 49
    coronal section, 24, 25
    sagittal section, 8, 9
  vestibulocochlear nerve of, 24, 25
Epiglottis
  axial section, 50, 51
  coronal section, 20, 21
  sagittal section, 4, 5

Esophagus, 172, 173
  axial section, 44–47, 54, 55, 58–69
  coronal section, 122, 123
  sagittal section, 108–111
Ethmoid sinuses, 4, 5
Eyes, 4, 5, 8–11
  eyelids, 6–9, 14
  lacrimal gland of, 8, 9
  lateral palpebral commissure, 10, 11
  lens of
    axial section, 44, 45
    coronal section, 14–16
    sagittal section, 8
  muscles of
    extrinsic ocular, 16, 17
    oblique, superior, 158
    rectus
      inferior, 6, 7, 158
      lateral, 44, 45
      medial, 44, 45, 158
      superior, 6, 7
  optic disc of, 44, 45
  retina of
    neural (detached), 14, 15, 44, 45
    pigmented layer of, 14, 15, 44, 45
  sclera
    axial section, 44, 45
    coronal section, 14–17
    sagittal section, 6–9
  vitreous of, 14, 16, 44, 45

Facial bones (Also see Cartilage)
  mandible. See Mandible
  maxilla
    axial section, 46, 47
    coronal section, 14–17
    sagittal section, 4, 5
  nasal, 44–47
  zygomatic
    axial section, 44–47
    coronal section, 14–17
    orbital part of, 44–47
    sagittal section, 8–11
Facial muscles
  buccinator muscle, 18, 19
  masseter muscle
    axial section, 48, 49
    coronal section, 16–19
    sagittal section, 10, 11
  temporalis muscle
    axial section, 42–47
    coronal section, 16–21
    sagittal section, 8–11
Facial nerve, 44–49
Fasciae
  prevertebral, 54, 55, 172, 173
  renal, 74, 75, 108, 109
  suprasternal space, 110, 111
  thoracolumbar, 84, 85, 94–97
Fat
  buccal pad
    coronal section, 14–17
    sagittal section, 10, 11
  infratemporal fossa, 16, 17
  ischiorectal fossa, 88, 89
  orbital, 6, 7, 44, 45
  pararenal fat body, 74, 75
  perinephric, 114
  periorbital, 14, 16
  renal pelvic, 76

Femur
  axial section, 86–91, 96, 97, 100, 101
  condyle of
    lateral, 140, 141, 144, 145
      medial, 144, 145
  coronal section, 122–125
  cross-section, 138, 139
  epiphyseal cartilage of, 144
  greater trochanter of
    axial section, 86, 87, 96, 97
    coronal section, 124, 125
    sagittal section, 104, 105, 116, 117
  head of, 140, 141
    axial section, 86, 87,
    coronal section, 122-125
    sagittal section, 106, 107, 116, 117
  intertrochanteric crest of, 88, 89
  lesser trochanter of, 122, 123, 140, 141
  longitudinal section, 140, 141, 144, 145
  neck of, 140, 141
    axial section, 96, 97
    coronal section, 122, 123
  ossification center for, 144
  sagittal section, 104–107, 116, 117
  trochanteric fossa, 88, 89
Fibula
  cross-section, 142, 143
  head of, 144, 145
  longitudinal section, 144, 145
  malleolus of, lateral, 144, 145
Finger, 136, 137
Fissures
  of brain. See Brain, fissures of
  of lung
    horizontal, 120, 121
      oblique, 62–67, 104–109, 114–117, 124,
      125
    transverse, 114, 115
Flocculus, 44, 45, 151, 153
Fonticulus
  anterior, 2–5, 18–25, 32–35, 158
  mastoid, 28, 29, 42, 43
  posterior, 2, 3
  sphenoid, 10, 11, 20, 21, 42, 43
Foot, 144, 146, 147
Forearm
  cross-section, 132, 133
  longitudinal section, 130, 131
Fossae
  cranial
    anterior, 18, 19, 40, 41, 44, 45
    middle, 10, 11, 18, 19, 40–45
    posterior, 26, 27, 44, 45
  infratemporal, 16, 17
  ischiorectal, 88, 89
  jugular, 24, 25, 46, 47
  ovalis, 170, 171
  trochanteric, 88, 89
Frontal bone
  axial section, 38–43
  coronal section, 14–19
  sagittal section, 2–11

Gallbladder
  axial section, 72-77
  sagittal section, 112, 113, 116
Ganglia
  dorsal spinal
    of C5 spinal nerve, 54, 55
    in intervertebral foramen, 60, 61
    of L3 spinal nerve, 76, 77
    of T4 spinal nerve, 62, 63

sympathetic
  of lumbar trunk, 78, 79
  superior, 50, 51
Gyri. See Brain, gyri of

Hand
  cross-section, 134, 135
  sagittal section, 106, 107
Hard palate
  axial section, 48, 49
  coronal section, 14–17
  sagittal section, 2–5
Heart
  aortic sinus of, 166, 167
  apex of, 164–167
    axial section, 64–69
    sagittal section, 104, 105
  atria of, 164–173
    auricle of, 164, 168–173
    axial section, 64, 65
    coronal section, 120, 121
    sagittal section, 108–113
  atrioventricular sulcus of, 164, 165
  axial section, 62–69
  chordae tendineae, 166-171
  coronal section, 120, 145
  coronary sinus of, 165, 168, 169, 170,
    171
    coronal section, 120, 121
    sagittal section, 110, 111
  coronary sulcus of, 164, 165
  ductus arteriosus, 164
    axial section, 62, 63
    sagittal section, 110, 111
  ductus venosus, 160, 161, 172, 173
    axial section, 66–69
    coronal section, 120, 121
    sagittal section, 112, 113
  foramen ovale of, 166, 167
  fossa ovalis, 170, 171
  interatrial septum, 64, 65, 166, 167
  interventricular septum of, 166–169
    axial section, 64, 65
    sagittal section, 110, 111
  interventricular sulcus of, 164, 165
  musculi pectinati, 166, 167
  papillary muscle, 166, 167, 170, 171
    axial section, 64, 65
    sagittal section, 108, 109
  sagittal section, 104–113
  septum primum of, 166, 167, 170, 171
  sinus venarum of, 170, 171
  trabeculae carneae, 166-171
  valves of
    aortic, 166, 167, 170, 171
    for foramen ovale, 166, 167
    mitral, 166-171
    tricuspid, 63, 65, 166-169
  ventricles of, 164–173
    axial section, 64–67
    coronal section, 120, 121
    sagittal section, 106–113
Hip
  acetabulum
    axial section, 86, 87
    coronal section, 122–125
    longitudinal section, 140, 141
    sagittal section, 106, 107, 116, 117
  ilium. See Ilium
  ischium
    axial section, 86, 87, 96, 97
    coronal section, 124, 125

    sagittal section, 108, 109
  pubis. See Pubis
Hippocampus
  axial section, 38–41
  coronal section, 22-27
  sagittal section, 6-9
Humerus
  anatomical neck of, 58, 59
  capitulum of, 130, 131
  coronal section, 120–123
  greater tubercle of, 58, 59
  head of, 58, 59
  lesser tubercle of, 58, 59
  longitudinal section, 130, 131
Hyoid bone
  axial section, 50, 51
  coronal section, 18-21
  sagittal section, 2-7
Hypothalamus, 2, 3

Ilium
  ala of
    axial section, 84, 85, 94, 95
    coronal section, 122–125
    sagittal section, 104-107, 116, 117
  auricular surface of, 108, 109, 114, 115
  body of, 124, 125
  coronal section, 122–125
  crest of
    coronal section, 124, 125
    sagittal section, 106, 107, 116, 117
  fossa of, 94, 95
  sagittal section, 106–109, 114–117
  spine of
    anterior superior, 84, 85
    posterior inferior, 108, 109, 114, 115
    posterior superior, 108, 109, 114, 115
  tuberosity of, 108, 109, 114, 115
Intercostal muscles
  axial section, 62, 63, 70, 71
  sagittal section, 106, 107
Intercostal nerves, 64, 65
Interosseous membrane
  antebrachial, 132, 133
  crural, 142-145
Intervertebral discs
  coronal section, 124, 125
  sagittal section, 110–113
Ischium
  axial section, 86, 87, 96, 97
  coronal section, 124, 125
  sagittal section, 108, 109

Jaws
  mandible. See Mandible
  maxilla
    axial section, 46, 47
    coronal section, 14–17
    sagittal section, 4, 5
Joints
  ankle, 144, 145
  atlanto-occipital, 2, 3, 6, 7
  calcaneocuboid, 146, 147
  costotransverse, 70, 71
  costovertebral, 60, 61, 64, 65
  cuboideometatarsal, 146, 147
  interphalangeal
    distal, 136, 137
    proximal, 136, 137
  knee
    capsule of, 140, 141

lateral meniscus of, 140, 141, 144, 145
  medial meniscus of, 144, 145
metatarsophalangeal, 146, 147
sacroiliac, 84, 85, 94, 95
sternoclavicular, 60, 61
temporomandibular, 20, 21
tibiofibular, 144, 145
Jugular bulb, 158
  axial section, 44, 45, 48, 49
  coronal section, 26–29
Jugular fossa, 24, 25, 46, 47

Kidney
  axial section, 74–79
  coronal section, 122–125
  cortex of, 76, 77
  fasciae around, 74, 75
  lobules of, 116, 117, 124, 125
  major calyx of, 76, 77
  medulla of, 76, 77
  pelvis of, 76, 77, 106, 107, 114, 115
  pyramid, renal, 114
  sagittal section, 104–109, 114–117
Knee
  capsule of, 140, 141
  lateral meniscus of, 140, 141, 144, 145
  medial meniscus of, 144, 145

Large intestine
  appendix, vermiform
    axial section, 78, 79
    sagittal section, 114, 115
  cecum, 80, 81
  colon
    ascending, 76–79, 124, 125
    colic flexure of, 122, 123
    descending, 74–81, 122, 123
    sigmoid, 110–113
    splenic flexure of, 104, 105
    transverse, 76-79, 106–113
Larynx
  arytenoid cartilage, 2, 3
  coronal section, 120, 121
  cricoarytenoid, posterior, muscle of, 54, 55
  cricoid cartilage, 52–55, 112, 113
  cricothyroid muscle of, 54, 55
  epiglottis, 4, 5, 20, 50, 51
  infraglottic cavity of, 54, 55
  laryngopharynx, 50–53
  rima glottidis, 52, 53
  thyroarytenoid muscle of, 52, 53
  thyroid cartilage, 6, 7, 20, 21, 50–55, 120, 145
  vocal fold (cord), 4, 5, 52, 53
Lens of eye
  axial section, 44, 45
  coronal section, 14–16
  sagittal section, 8
Ligaments
  anococcygeal, 90, 91, 100, 101
  of atlas, transverse, 50, 51
  calcaneofibular, 144, 145
  calcaneonavicular, 146, 147
  coracoclavicular, 116, 117
  cruciate, anterior, 144, 145
  denticulate, 54, 55, 58, 59
  falciform, 70–77
  of femur head, 86, 87, 96, 97
  fibular collateral, 144, 145
  ligamentum nuchae, 50–55, 112, 113

pubic, arcuate, 88, 89
round, of uterus, 94, 95
sacrococcygeal, 86, 87
  deep dorsal, 88, 89
  deep posterior, 98, 99
sacroiliac, interosseous, 84, 85
sacrotuberous, 98, 99, 108, 109
tibial collateral, 144, 145
tibiotalar part of medial (deltoid), 144, 145
Lines
  linea alba, 78, 79
  semilunar, 78, 79, 120, 121
Lips
  axial section, 48, 49
  coronal section, 16
  sagittal section, 6-9
Liver
  axial section, 66–77
  coronal section, 120–125
  hepatic duct, common, 72, 73
  lobes of, 160, 161, 172, 173
    caudate, 68–73, 110, 111, 160, 161, 172, 173
    quadrate, 74–77, 112, 113
  sagittal section, 104–114, 116, 117
Lungs
  bronchi of, 172, 173
    axial section, 62, 63
    coronal section, 122, 123
    sagittal section, 108–113
  coronal section, 120–125
  horizontal fissure of, 120, 121
  inferior lobe of
    axial section, 62–69
    coronal section, 124, 125
    sagittal section, 104, 105, 108, 109, 112–117
  middle lobe of, 64–67, 114–117
  oblique fissure of
    axial section, 62–67
    coronal section, 124, 125
    sagittal section, 104–109, 114–117
  sagittal section, 104–117
  superior lobe of
    axial section, 58, 60–67
    coronal section, 120–125
    sagittal section, 104–109, 114, 115
  superior lobe of, 172, 173
  transverse fissure of, 114, 115
Lymph nodes, cervical, 50, 51

Mandible, 158
  axial section, 48-51
  body of, 2, 3, 6, 7, 18, 19
  condylar process of, 10, 11, 20, 21
  coronal section, 14–21
  coronoid process of, 48, 49
  neck of, 18, 19, 48, 49
  ramus of, 8, 9
  sagittal section, 2–9
  symphysis of, 50, 51
  temporomandibular joint, 20, 21
Maxilla
  axial section, 46, 47
  coronal section, 14–17
  sagittal section, 4, 5
Mediastinum
  pericardium of, 66, 67, 106, 107
  pleura of, 66–69
Membranes
  atlanto-occipital, 28, 29

interosseous
  antebrachial, 132, 133
  crural, 142–145
  obturator, 88, 89, 98, 99
  tympanic, 22, 23, 46–49
Metacarpal bones,
  cross-section, 134, 135
  longitudinal section, 136, 137
  ossification center of, 133–137
Metatarsal bones, 146, 147
Mouth. See Oral cavity
Muscles
  abductor digiti brevis, 134, 135
  abductor hallucis, 146, 147
  abductor pollicis brevis, 134, 135
  adductor brevis
    axial section, 88, 89, 96, 97
    cross-section, 138, 139
    sagittal section, 106, 107
  adductor hallucis, 146, 147
  adductor longus
    axial section, 96, 97
    cross-section, 138, 139
    sagittal section, 106, 107
  adductor magnus
    axial section, 88, 89, 96, 97
    coronal section, 122, 123
    cross-section, 138, 139
    longitudinal section, 140, 141
    sagittal section, 106, 107
  adductor pollicis, 134, 135
  biceps brachii, 58, 59
  biceps femoris, 90, 91, 98–101
    coronal section, 124, 125
    cross-section, 138, 139
    longitudinal section, 140, 141
  brachialis, 130, 131
  brachioradialis, 130, 131
  buccinator, 18, 19
  bulbospongiosus, 90, 91
  coccygeus, 112–115
  coracobrachialis, 58, 59
  craniovertebral, deep, 2–9
  cricoarytenoid, posterior, 54, 55
  cricothyroid, 54, 55
  deltoid, 58, 59, 120, 145
  digastric
    anterior belly of, 14–17
    posterior belly of, 10, 11, 50, 51
  erector spinae
    axial section, 74–81, 84, 85, 94, 95
    sagittal section, 106, 107, 114, 115
  extensor carpi ulnaris, 132, 133
  extensor digiti minimi, 132, 133
  extensor digitorum, 132, 133
  extensor digitorum longus, 142, 143
  extensor hallucis longus, 142, 143
  extensor indicis, 132, 133
  extensor pollicis brevis, 132, 133
  extensor pollicis longus, 132, 133
  flexor carpi ulnaris, 132, 133
  flexor digiti minimi brevis, 134, 135
  flexor digitorum longus, 142, 143
  flexor digitorum profundus, 132, 133
  flexor digitorum superficialis, 132, 133
  flexor hallucis brevis, 146, 147
  flexor pollicis longus, 132, 133
  gastrocnemius
    cross-section, 142, 143
    longitudinal section, 140, 141
  gemellus
    inferior, 140, 141
    superior, 96, 97

Muscles (*cont.*)
  genioglossus
    coronal section, 14–17
    sagittal section, 2–5
  geniohyoid
    axial section, 50, 51
    coronal section, 14–17
    sagittal section, 2–5
  gluteus maximus
    axial section, 84–91, 94-101
    coronal section, 122–125
    cross-section, 138, 139
    sagittal section, 104–109, 114–117
  gluteus medius
    axial section, 84–87, 94–97
    coronal section, 122–125
    sagittal section, 104–107, 116, 117
  gluteus minimus
    axial section, 96, 97
    coronal section, 122–125
    sagittal section, 104–107, 116, 117
  gracilis
    axial section, 96, 97
    cross-section, 138, 139
  hyoglossus, 50, 51
  iliacus
    coronal section, 124, 125
    sagittal section, 116, 117
  iliocostalis lumborum
    axial section, 70–73
    sagittal section, 116, 117
  iliocostalis thoracis, 62-69
  iliopsoas
    axial section, 84, 85, 94, 95
    coronal section, 122, 123
    sagittal section, 104–107
  infrahyoid, 172, 173
  infraspinatus
    axial section, 58–61
    coronal section, 122–125
    longitudinal section, 130
  intercostal
    axial section, 62, 63, 70, 71
    sagittal section, 106, 107
  interosseous
    dorsal, 134, 135, 146, 147
    palmar, 134, 135
    plantar, 146, 147
  ischiocavernous, 90, 91
  latissimus dorsi, 172, 173
    axial section, 64–77
    coronal section, 120–123
    sagittal section, 104, 105
  levator ani
    arcus tendineus of, 114, 115
    axial section, 86, 87, 98, 99
    coronal section, 124, 125
    sagittal section, 108, 109, 112–115
  levator scapulae
    axial section, 52–55, 58, 59
    sagittal section, 106, 107
  longissimus thoracis
    axial section, 62–73
    sagittal section, 114, 115
  longus capitis
    axial section, 46–55
    coronal section, 22, 23
  longus colli
    axial section, 52–55, 58, 59
    coronal section, 112, 113
    sagittal section, 2, 3
  lumbrical, 134–137

  masseter
    axial section, 48, 49
    coronal section, 16–19
    sagittal section, 10, 11
  multifidi
    axial section, 52–55, 58-81, 84, 85, 94–97
    coronal section, 124, 125
  mylohyoid
    axial section, 50, 51, 54, 55
    coronal section, 14–17
  oblique abdominal, external
    axial section, 74-81, 84, 85
    coronal section, 122–125
    sagittal section, 104, 105
  oblique abdominal, internal
    axial section, 72, 73, 79–85
    coronal section, 122–125
    sagittal section, 104, 105, 116, 117
  oblique muscle of eye, superior, 158
  obturator externus
    axial, 88, 89, 98, 99
    coronal section, 122, 123
    sagittal section, 106-109, 114, 115
  obturator internus
    axial section, 86–89, 96–99
    sagittal section, 108, 109, 114, 115
  ocular, extrinsic, 16, 17
  omohyoid
    axial section, 52, 53, 58, 59
    inferior belly, 106–109
    sagittal section, 106–109
  opponens digiti minimi, 134, 135
  opponens pollicis, 134, 135
  orbicularis oris, 8, 9
  pectineus
    axial section, 86, 87, 96, 97
    sagittal section, 106, 107, 114, 115
  pectoralis major
    axial section, 58–63
    sagittal section, 104–107, 114–117
  pectoralis minor
    axial section, 58–63
    sagittal section, 104, 105, 116, 117
  peroneus (fibularis) brevis, 142–145
  peroneus (fibularis) longus, 142–145
  pharyngeal constrictor, inferior, 50–53
  piriformis
    axial section, 88, 89, 96, 97
    sagittal section, 108, 109, 114, 115
  platysma, 8, 9
  pronator quadratus, 132, 133
  pronator teres, 130, 131
  psoas major
    axial section, 76–81
    coronal section, 124, 125
    sagittal section, 108, 109, 112–115
  pterygoid
    lateral, 18, 19, 46, 47
    medial, 18, 19, 48, 49
  quadratus femoris, 124, 125, 140, 141
  quadratus lumborum
    axial section, 74–81, 96, 97
    sagittal section, 106, 107, 114, 115
  quadratus plantae, 146, 147
  rectus muscles of eye
    inferior, 6, 7, 158
    lateral, 44, 45
    medial, 44, 45, 158
    superior, 6, 7
  rectus abdominis
    axial section, 70-81, 84, 85, 94, 95
    coronal section, 120, 121

    sagittal section, 114, 115
  rectus capitis posterior major, 46, 47
  rectus capitis posterior minor, 50, 51
  rectus femoris
    axial section, 86, 87, 94, 95
    coronal section, 122, 123
    cross-section, 138, 139
    longitudinal section, 140, 141
    sagittal section, 104, 105, 116, 117
  rhomboideus major, 172, 173
    axial section, 62, 63
    sagittal section, 106, 107, 114, 115
  sartorius
    axial section, 86, 87, 94, 95
    cross-section, 138, 139
    longitudinal section, 140, 141
  scalene
    anterior, 52–55, 58, 59, 122, 123
    middle, 52, 55, 58, 59
    posterior, 54, 55, 58, 59
  semimembranous, 138, 139
  semispinalis capitis
    axial section, 44–47, 50–55, 58–61
    coronal section, 30
    sagittal section, 114, 115
  semispinalis cervicis, 58-61
  semispinalis thoracis, 62-67
  semitendinosus
    axial section, 90, 91, 98-101
    coronal section, 122–125
    cross-section, 138, 139
    longitudinal section, 140, 141
    sagittal section, 106, 107
  serratus anterior
    axial section, 60-69
    coronal section, 120–125
    sagittal section, 104, 105, 116, 117
  serratus posterior inferior
    axial section, 70, 71
    sagittal section, 106, 107
  serratus posterior superior, 58, 59
  soleus, 142-145
  spinalis cervicis, 54, 55
  splenius capitis
    axial section, 50–55, 58–61
    sagittal section, 108, 109, 114, 115
  stapedius, 46, 47
  sternocleidomastoid
    axial section, 50-55, 58, 59
    coronal section, 26, 27, 120, 121
    sagittal section, 10, 11, 112–115
  sternohyoid
    axial section, 52–55, 58, 59
    sagittal section, 108, 109
  sternothyroid, 52–55, 58, 59
  stylohyoid, 8-11
  subclavius
    axial section, 58, 59
    sagittal section, 104–107
  subscapularis
    axial section, 58–63
    coronal section, 120–125
    longitudinal section, 130
    sagittal section, 104, 105
  supraspinatus
    axial section, 58, 59
    coronal section, 124, 125
    longitudinal section, 130
    sagittal section, 104, 105, 116, 117
  temporalis
    axial section, 42-47
    coronal section, 16-21

sagittal section, 8-11
tensor fasciae latae, 86, 87, 94-97
teres major
  axial section, 62, 63
  coronal section, 120, 145
thyroarytenoid, 52, 53
tibialis anterior, 142, 143
tibialis posterior, 142, 143
transverse abdominal
  axial section, 72, 73, 79–85
  sagittal section, 104, 105
  coronal section, 122–125
trapezius, 172, 173
  axial section, 44–55, 58–67
  coronal section, 124, 125
  sagittal section, 104–109, 114–117
triceps brachii
  coronal section, 120, 121
  longitudinal section, 130, 131
urethral sphincter, of urogenital diaphragm, 98, 99
vaginal sphincter, of urogenital diaphragm, 98, 99
vastus intermedius, 138–141
vastus lateralis
  axial section, 88, 89
  coronal section, 122, 123
  cross-section, 138, 139
  sagittal section, 104, 105
vastus medialis, 138, 139

Nail, 136, 137
Nasopharynx
  axial section, 46–49
  coronal section of, 18–21
  sagittal section, 2, 3
Neck
  atlas. *See* Atlas
  axis of. *See* Axis
  esophagus in, 172, 173
  axial section, 44–47, 54, 55, 58–69
  coronal section, 122, 123
  sagittal section, 108–111
  hyoid bone of
    axial section, 50, 51
    coronal section, 18–21
    sagittal section, 2–7
  larynx in. *See* Larynx
  muscles of
    craniovertebral muscles of, 2, 3
    digastric, 10, 11, 14–17, 50, 51
    geniohyoid, 2–5, 14–17, 50, 51
    longus capitis, 22, 23, 46–55
    longus colli muscle, 2, 3, 52–55, 58,
      59, 112, 113
    multifidi, 52–55, 58-81, 84, 85, 94–97,
      124–125
    mylohyoid, 14–17, 50, 51, 54, 55
    omohyoid, 52, 53, 58, 59, 106–109
    platysma, 8, 9
    rectus capitis posterior major, 46, 47
    rectus capitis posterior minor, 50, 51
    scalene, 52–55, 58, 59, 122, 123
    semispinalis capitis, 30, 44–47, 50–55,
      58–61, 114, 115
    spinalis cervicis, 54, 55
    splenius capitis, 50–55, 58–61, 108,
      109, 114, 115
    sternocleidomastoid, 10, 11, 26, 27,
      50–55, 58, 59, 112–115, 120, 121
    sternohyoid, 52–55, 58, 59, 108, 109

sternothyroid, 52–55, 58, 59
stylohyoid, 8–11
pharynx. *See* Pharnyx
thymus gland, 172, 173
  axial section, 60–63
  coronal section, 120, 121
  sagittal section, 110–113
thyroid gland, 54, 55, 58, 59
trachea
  axial section, 58–61
  coronal section, 122, 123
  sagittal section, 110–113
Nerve plexus
  brachial, 60, 61, 104, 105
  sacral, 84, 85, 94, 95
Nerves
  abducens, 20, 21, 44, 45
  alveolar, inferior, 16, 17
  cochlear, 6, 7
  facial nerve, 44–49
  femoral, 84, 85, 122, 123
  fibular (peroneal), superficial, 142,
    143
  ganglion. *See* Ganglia
  intercostal, 64, 65
  lumbosacral trunk, 108, 109, 112–115
  mandibular, 46, 47
  maxillary, 20, 21
  median, 132–135
  obturator, 96, 97, 108, 109, 114, 115
  oculomotor nerve, 2–5, 20–23, 42,
    43
  ophthalmic, 20, 21
  optic, 2-5, 44, 45, 151
  of penis, dorsal, 88, 89
  phrenic, 64, 65
  plexuses of. *See* Nerve plexus
  sciatic
    axial section, 86–89, 96–99
    coronal section, 122, 123
    cross-section, 138, 139
    longitudinal section, 140, 141
    sagittal section, 108, 109
  spinal. *See* Spinal nerves
  tibial, 142, 143
  trochlear, 20, 21
  ulnar, 132–135
  vagus, 50–55, 58–61
  vestibulocochlear, 24, 25
Nose
  cartilage of, lateral, 44–47
  cavity of, 44–47
  choana, 46, 47
  coronal section, 14–17
  inferior concha
    coronal section, 14–17
    sagittal section, 4, 5
  inferior meatus, 4, 5
  middle concha, 14-17, 46, 47
  middle meatus, 46, 47
  naris, 4, 5
  sagittal section, 2–7
  septum of
    axial section, 44–47
    coronal section, 14–17
    sagittal section, 2, 3
  sphenoid concha, 18, 19

Occipital bone
  axial section, 34–49
  basilar part, 2–5, 22, 23, 44–49

coronal section, 22, 23, 26-30
  lateral part, 2–5, 8–11, 28, 29, 38, 39,
    44–49, 158
  sagittal section, 2–5, 8–11
  squamous part, 2-5, 8-11, 30, 34-37, 40-
    43, 158
Omentum
  greater, 112, 113
  lesser, 70, 71, 110, 111
Oral cavity
  axial section, 48–51
  buccal fat pad
    coronal section, 14–17
    sagittal section, 10, 11
  coronal section, 14–19
  gingiva, 14, 15, 48, 49
  lips, 6–9, 16, 48, 49
  oropharynx
    coronal section, 20–23
    sagittal section, 2–5
  parotid gland, 46–49
  submandibular gland
    axial section, 50, 51
    coronal section, 14, 15, 18, 19
  teeth. *See* Teeth
  tongue, 158
    axial section, 50, 51
    coronal section, 14–19
    sagittal section, 2–7
  uvula, 44, 45, 48, 49
Orbit
  axial section, 44, 45
  coronal section, 14, 15
  fat of, 6, 7, 14, 16, 44, 45
  inferior fissure of, 46, 47
  roof of, 158
Oropharynx
  coronal section, 20–23
  sagittal section, 2–5

Palate
  hard
    axial section, 48, 49
    coronal section, 14–17
    sagittal section, 2–5
  soft
    axial section, 48, 49
    coronal section, 18, 19
    sagittal section, 2–5
Pancreas
  axial section, 72–75
  body of, 72, 73, 106, 107
  coronal section, 122, 123
  head of, 74, 75, 110, 111, 122, 123, 160,
    161, 172, 173
  neck of, 108, 109
  sagittal section, 104–111
  tail of, 72, 73, 104, 105
Paranasal sinuses
  ethmoid sinuses, 4, 5
  maxillary sinus, 14, 15
Parietal bone
  axial section, 32–35, 38–43
  coronal section, 20–24, 26, 28, 29
  sagittal section, 2–11
Peduncles
  cerebellar, 24, 25
    middle, 26, 27, 42, 43
    superior, 2, 3, 26, 27
  cerebral, 150
    axial section, 40–43

Peduncles (*cont.*)
　　coronal section, 24, 25
　　sagittal section, 108, 109
Pericardial cavity, 66–69, 172, 173
Pericardium
　　axial section, 66, 67
　　sagittal section, 106, 107
Peritoneal cavity, 68, 69, 78, 79
Phalanx
　　of index finger, 134–137
　　of toe, 146, 147
Pharynx
　　laryngopharynx, 50–53
　　median raphe of, 48, 49
　　nasopharynx
　　　axial section, 46, 47
　　　coronal section, 18–21
　　　sagittal section, 2–5
　　oropharynx
　　　coronal section, 20–23
　　　sagittal section, 2–5
　　palatopharyngeal arch of, 48, 49
　　passavant fold or ridge of, 20, 21
　　pharyngeal constrictor muscle of, inferior, 50–53
　　retropharyngeal space, 50, 51
Pituitary gland, 2–5
Plexus, *See* Nerve plexus
Pleura, 66, 67
Pleural cavity, 60–69
Pons, 150, 151, 153
　　axial section, 42–45
　　sagittal section, 2, 4, 5
Pubis
　　axial section, 86–89, 96, 97
　　body of, 86, 87
　　coronal section, 122, 123
　　inferior ramus of, 98, 99, 112–115
　　sagittal section, 108–115
　　superior ramus of, 86, 87, 108, 109, 112–115
　　symphysis of, 86, 87, 96, 97, 122, 123

Radius
　　cross-section, 132–135
　　distal end of, 136, 137
　　head of, 130, 131
　　longitudinal section, 130, 131, 136, 137
　　neck of, 130, 131
Rectum
　　axial section, 80, 81, 84–99
　　coronal section, 124, 125
　　sagittal section, 110, 111
　　transverse rectal fold, 88, 89, 98, 99
Reproductive system, female
　　cervix, 96, 97
　　clitoris, 98, 99
　　clitoris, 122, 123
　　labial commissures, 96, 97, 100, 101
　　labium majus, 98, 99, 100, 101
　　labium minus, 98, 99
　　rectouterine pouch, 94, 95
　　uterus, 94, 95
　　vagina, 96–99
　　vesicouterine pouch, 94, 95
Reproductive system, male
　　dartos tunic, 90, 91
　　falx inguinalis, 86, 87
　　gubernaculum, 84, 85
　　penis, 88–91
　　　corpus cavernosum of, 88, 89
　　　corpus spongiosum of, 88, 89

　　dorsal artery of, 88, 89
　　dorsal nerve of, 88, 89
　　sagittal section, 108, 109
　　tunica albuginea of, 88, 89
　processus vaginalis, 84, 85
　prostate gland
　　axial section, 88, 89
　　sagittal section, 110, 111
　scrotum
　　axial section, 90, 91
　　sagittal section, 108, 109
　seminal vesicle, 110, 111
　testes, 90, 91
　utricle, prostatic, 88, 89
Retina of eye
　neural (detached), 14, 15, 44, 45
　pigmented layer of, 14, 15, 44, 45
Ribs
　1st, 58, 60, 61, 106–109, 114–117, 124, 125
　2nd, 60, 61, 104, 105
　3rd, 62, 63, 104, 105, 116, 117
　4th, 62–65, 108, 109
　5th, 66, 67
　6th, 106, 107, 114, 115
　7th, 68, 69, 120, 121
　8th, 64, 65, 68–71, 122, 123
　9th, 66–93, 108, 109, 116
　10th, 68–73, 124, 125
　11th, 70–77, 104, 105
　12th, 72–77, 104–109, 116, 117

Sacral canal, 84–87, 110, 111
Sacrum
　anterior foramen of, 94, 95
　axial section, 84-87, 94–97
　coronal section, 124, 125
　dorsal part of, 84, 85, 94–97
　hiatus of, 98, 99, 110, 111
　lateral part of, 84–87, 94–97
　posterior foramen of, 94, 95
　sagittal section, 110–113
Salivary glands
　parotid gland, 46–49
　submandibular gland, 158
　　axial section, 50, 51
　　coronal section, 14, 15, 18, 19
Scapula
　acromion of, 58, 59, 120, 121
　axial section, 58–63
　body of, 104, 105, 130
　coracoid process of, 58, 59, 116, 117
　coronal section, 120–125, 145
　glenoid cavity of, 58, 59, 120, 121
　glenoid labrum of, 58, 59
　longitudinal section, 130
　neck of, 58, 59
　sagittal section, 104, 105, 116, 117
　spine of, 58, 59, 104, 105, 122–125
Septum
　interatrial, 166, 167
　interventricular, 166–169
　nasal
　　axial section, 44–47
　　coronal section, 16, 17
　　sagittal section, 2, 3
　pellucidum
　　axial section, 38, 39
　　cavum of, 156
　　coronal section, 18, 20, 21
　　lamina of, 154, 155
　　sagittal section, 4, 5
　primum, 166, 167, 170, 171

Sinuses
　of brain. *See* Brain, sinuses of
　of heart
　　aortic, 166, 167
　　coronary, 165, 168, 169, 170, 171
　　　coronal section, 120, 121
　　　sagittal section, 110, 111
　　venarum, 170, 171
　paranasal
　　ethmoid sinuses, 4, 5
　　maxillary sinus, 14, 15
Skull
　clinoid process, 22, 23
　cranial fossa
　　anterior, 18, 19, 40, 41, 44, 45
　　middle, 10, 11, 18, 19, 40–45
　　posterior, 26, 27, 44, 45
　crista galli, 2, 3, 14, 15, 158
　facial canal, 26, 27
　foramen magnum, 2, 3, 24, 25, 48, 49
　frontal bone
　　axial section, 38–43
　　coronal section, 14–19
　　sagittal section, 2–11
　hard palate
　　axial section, 48, 49
　　coronal section, 14–17
　　sagittal section, 2–5
　jugular fossa of, 24, 25, 46, 47
　mastoid antrum, 44, 45
　nasoethmoid complex, 44, 45
　nasolacrimal duct of, 46, 47
　occipital bone. *See* Occipital bone
　orbit. *See* Orbit
　parietal bone. *See* Parietal bone
　sella turcica, 44, 45
　sphenoid bone. *See* Sphenoid bone
　sutures of
　　coronal, 6, 7, 36–41
　　frontal, 2, 3, 14–17, 36–43
　　lambdoidal, 34–43
　　occipitomastoid, 28, 29
　　sagittal, 2, 3, 26–30, 32, 33
　　sphenosquamosal, 44, 45
　　sphenozygomatic, 44, 45
　　squamosal, 22, 23
　　temporozygomatic, 46, 47
　synchondrosis of, spheno-occipital, 2, 3
　tegmen tympani, 10, 11
　temporal bone. *See* Temporal bone
　zygomatic bone
　　axial section, 44–47
　　coronal section, 14–17
　　orbital part of, 44–47
　　sagittal section, 8–11
Small intestine
　duodenojejunal flexure of, 122, 123
　duodenum, 160, 161, 172, 173
　　axial section, 74–77
　　coronal section, 122, 123
　　sagittal section, 108–113
　ileum
　　axial section, 78–81
　　coronal section, 120–123
　　sagittal section, 106–109, 112–115
　jejunum, 160, 161, 172, 173
　　axial section, 74–77
　　coronal section, 120–123
　　sagittal section, 104–113
　mesentery of
　　axial section, 76–79
　　sagittal section, 112, 113

Soft palate
  axial section, 48, 49
  coronal section, 18, 19
  sagittal section, 2–5
Sphenoid bone
  axial section, 44–47
  body of, 20–21, 44, 45
  coronal section, 18–21
  greater wing of, 8, 9, 44, 45, 158
  lesser wing of, 158
  pterygoid process of, 18, 19, 46, 47
  sagittal section, 2, 3, 6–9
Spinal medulla (cord)
  axial section, 50–55, 58–79
  cervical, 50–55
  coronal section, 26, 27, 124, 125
  dura mater of, 58, 59, 110, 111, 124, 125
  sagittal section, 4, 5, 110, 111
  subarachnoid space of, 58–61
  thoracic, 58–79
Spinal nerves
  C4, 114, 115
  C5, 112, 113, 172, 173
  C6, 172, 173
  C7, 172, 173
  C8, 112, 113, 172, 173
  L2, 112, 113
  L3, 76, 77
  S1, 124, 125
  S2, 84, 85, 94, 95
  T2, 60, 61
  T4, 62, 63
  T7, 110, 111
  T8, 64, 65
  T10, 172, 173
Spleen
  axial section, 70–73
  coronal section, 120–125
  sagittal section, 104–107
Sternum
  axial section, 60–63, 68, 69
  body of, 62–65, 110–113
  cartilaginous, 172, 173
  manubrium of, 60, 61, 110–113, 172, 173
  sagittal section, 110–113
  xiphoid process of, 66–69, 110, 111, 172, 173
Stomach
  axial section, 70–73
  coronal section, 120–123
  sagittal section, 104–111
Sulci
  of brain. *See* Brain, sulci of
  of heart
    atrioventricular, 164, 165
    coronary, 164, 165
    interventricular, 164, 165
Suprarenal gland
  axial section, 70–75
  coronal section, 122–125
  sagittal section, 104–109, 112–115
Synchondroses
  between basilar and lateral parts of occipital bone, 46-49
  spheno-occipital, 2, 3, 22, 23, 44, 45

Talus, 144, 145
Teeth
  canine
    mandibular deciduous, 14, 15, 50, 51
    maxillary deciduous, 14, 15, 48, 49, 158

incisors
  first deciduous, 2-5
  mandibular deciduous, 50, 51
  maxillary deciduous, 48, 49
  second deciduous, 4, 5
molar
  first deciduous, 6, 7
  mandibular deciduous, 50, 51
  maxillary deciduous, 48, 49, 158
  second deciduous, 6, 7, 16, 17
Temporal bone
  axial section, 44–49
  coronal section, 18–29
  mandibular fossa of, 20, 21
  petrous part of, 10, 11, 22–25, 44, 45, 158
  sagittal section, 10, 11
  squamous part of, 10, 11, 20–23, 44, 45
  zygomatic process of, 18, 19, 46, 47
Tendons
  of brachioradialis muscle, 132, 133
  of extensor carpi radialis longus and brevis muscles, 132, 133
  of extensor digiti minimi muscle, 134, 135
  of extensor digitorum muscle, 134–137
  of flexor carpi radialis muscle, 132, 133
  of flexor digitorum profundus muscles, 134-137
  of flexor digitorum superficialis muscles, 134-137
  of flexor pollicis longus muscle, 134, 135
  of palmaris longus muscle, 132, 133
  perineal, central, 90, 91, 98-101
  of peroneus (fibularis) longus muscle, 146, 147
  of popliteus muscle, 144, 145
Thalamus, 154, 155
  axial section, 38–41
  coronal section, 22–27
  sagittal section, 2–7
Thigh
  cross-section, 138, 139
  femur. *See* Femur
  longitudinal section, 140, 141
Thoracic duct
  axial section, 60, 61, 68–73
  cisterna chyli, 72, 73
Thymus gland, 172, 173
  axial section, 60–63
  coronal section, 120, 121
  sagittal section, 110–113
Thyroid gland
  axial section, 54, 55
  isthmus of, 58, 59
  lateral lobe of, 58, 59
Tibia
  condyle of
    lateral, 140, 141, 144, 145
    medial, 144, 145
  cross-section, 142, 143
  epiphyseal cartilage of, 144
  intercondylar eminence of, 144, 145
  longitudinal section, 140, 141, 144, 145
  malleolus of, medial, 144, 145
  ossification center, 144
Tongue, 158
  axial section, 50, 51
  coronal section, 14–19
  sagittal section, 2–7
Tooth. *See* Teeth

Trachea
  axial section, 58–61
  coronal section, 122, 123
  sagittal section, 110–113
Turbinates. *See* Conchae

Ulna
  cross-section, 132–135
  longitudinal section, 130, 131
  olecranon of, 130, 131
Umbilical cord
  axial section, 80, 81, 84, 85
  sagittal section, 108–111
Ureters, 78–81, 84–87, 94, 95
Urethra
  female, 98, 99
  male, 88, 89

Vallecula, 20, 21
Valves of heart
  aortic, 166, 167, 170, 171
  for foramen ovale, 166, 167
  mitral, 166–171
  tricuspid, 166–169
Veins
  antebranchial, median, 132–135
  axillary
    coronal section, 122, 123
    sagittal section, 104, 105
  azygos, 170, 171
    axial section, 68–71
    coronal section, 122, 123
    sagittal section, 112, 113
  basilar, 26, 27, 132, 133
  brachiocephalic
    axial section, 60–63
    coronal section, 122, 123
    sagittal section, 110–113
  cardiac, 165, 166, 167
  cephalic, 132, 133
  cerebral
    great, 26, 27, 38–40, 158
    internal, 22–25, 38, 39, 154, 155
    superficial middle, 14, 15, 18, 19
  femoral, 86, 87, 138, 139
  fibular (peroneal), 142, 143
  gluteal, inferior, 86, 87
  hemiazygous, 68–71
  hepatic, 68, 69, 112, 120, 121
  iliac
    common, 80, 81
    external, 84, 85, 94, 95, 122, 123
    internal, 84, 85, 94, 95
  jugular
    external, 54, 55, 58, 59
    internal, 50–55, 58, 59
  maxillary, 10, 11
  of dorsal venous plexus of hand, 132–135
  portal, 160, 161
    axial section, 70–73
    coronal section, 120, 121
    sagittal section, 112, 113
  pudendal, internal, 88, 89
  pulmonary, 164–167, 172, 173
    coronal section, 122, 123
    sagittal section, 108, 109, 112, 113
  rectal, superior, 80, 81
  saphenous, greater, 138, 139, 142, 143
  subclavian, 106–109, 114, 115
  suprarenal, 160, 161

Veins (*cont.*)
  thyroid, inferior, 54, 55
  tibial, posterior, 142, 143
  umbilical, 160, 161
    axial section, 72, 76–79, 84, 85
    sagittal section, 112, 113
  vertebral, 58, 59
  vertebral venous plexus, anterior internal, 52-55
Vena cava
  inferior, 160, 161, 165, 170–173
    axial section, 66–79
    coronal section, 120, 121
    sagittal section, 112, 113
  superior, 164, 165, 170–173
    axial section, 62, 63
    sagittal section, 112, 113
Ventricles of brain
  fourth
    axial section, 42–45
    coronal section, 26, 27
    sagittal section, 2, 3
  lateral
    anterior horn of, 154, 156, 157

atrium of, 154-157
    axial section, 36–43
    body of, 154
    coronal section, 18–30
    lateral wall of, 154
    medial wall of, 154
    posterior horn of, 154, 155
    sagittal section, 2, 3, 6–9
  third
    axial section, 38–41
    coronal section, 20–25
Ventricles of heart
  axial section, 64–67
  coronal section, 120, 121
  sagittal section, 106–113
Vertebrae
  C2, 124, 125
  C3, 4, 5
    axial section, 52, 53
    body of, 52, 53
    lamina of, 52, 53
    ossification center of, 24, 25
    spinous process of, 52–55
  C4, 54, 55

C5, 54, 55, 112, 113
  C6, 58, 59, 122, 123
  C7, 120, 121
  L1, 72, 73, 112, 113, 172, 173
  L2, 74, 75, 112, 113
  L3, 76, 77
  L4, 78, 79
  L5, 80, 81, 110, 111, 124, 125
  T1, 58, 108, 109, 114, 115
  T2, 60, 61, 110, 111, 172, 173
  T4, 62, 63, 108, 109
  T8, 64, 65
  T9, 66, 67
  T10, 68, 69
  T11, 70, 71
  T12, 110, 111
  Vocal folds (cords) 4, 5, 52, 53

Zygomatic bone
  axial section, 44–47
  coronal section, 14–17
  orbital part of, 44–47
  sagittal section, 8–11

To the Community Library,

Thank you for the many hours of happiness my family has found within your walls. Happy Daydreaming!

Christine Gardner

A Moment of Quiet is Nothing to Fear

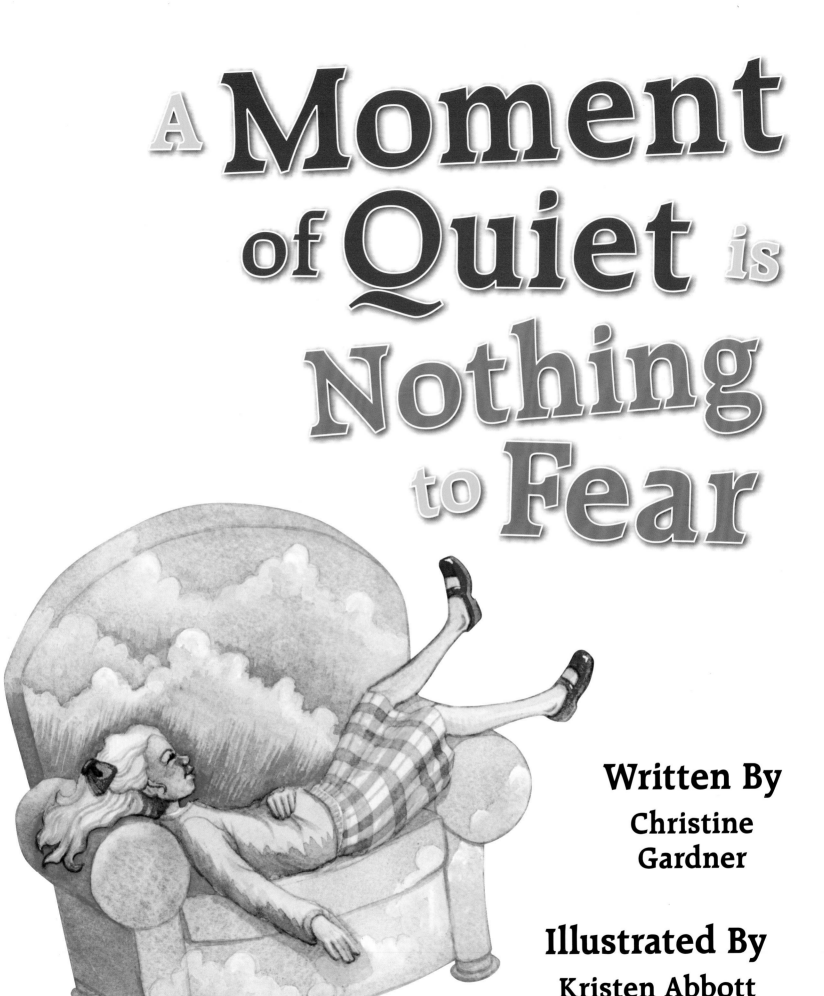

Written By

Christine
Gardner

Illustrated By

Kristen Abbott

Printed in Canada on a blend of 60%
post-consumer recycled and FSC certified paper.

Library of Congress Control Number: 2008908695
ISBN-13: 978-0-9821205-0-7

Published by:

moregreenmoms

www.moregreenmoms.com
2261 Jackson Street
San Francisco, CA 94115
415-346-9363

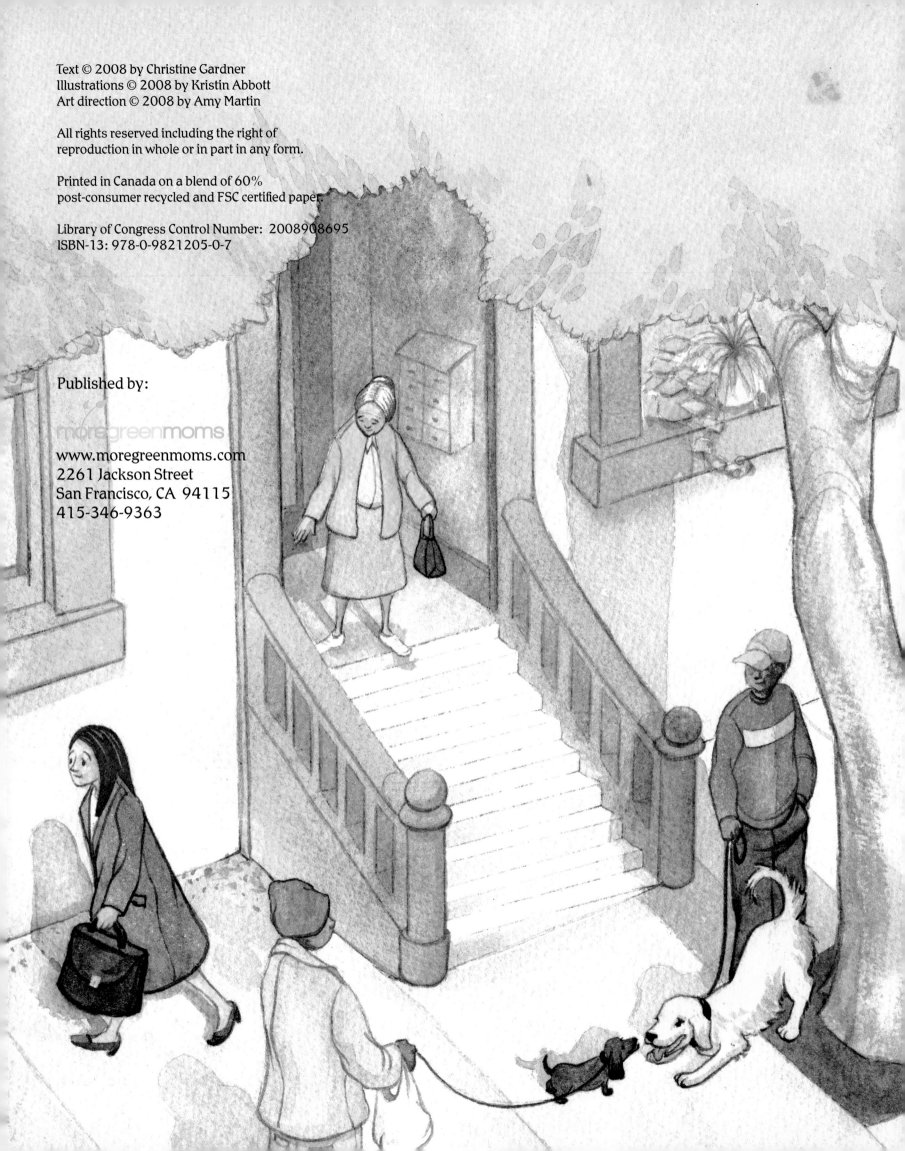

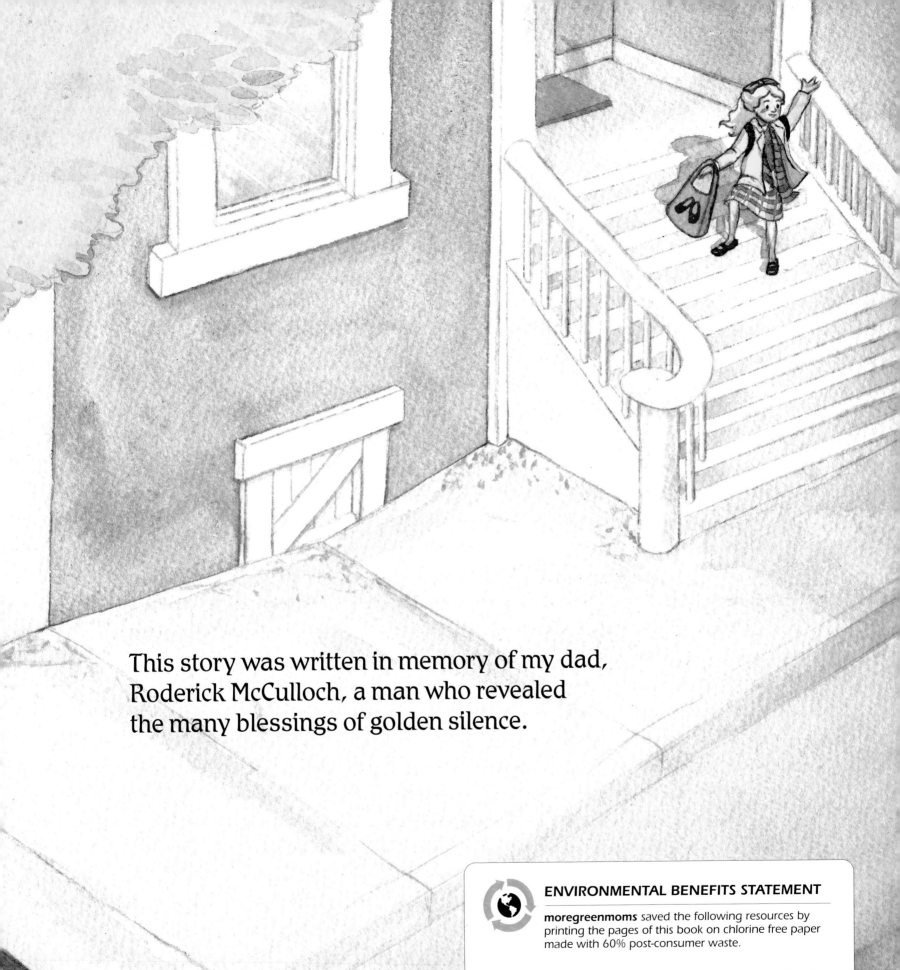

This story was written in memory of my dad,
Roderick McCulloch, a man who revealed
the many blessings of golden silence.

ENVIRONMENTAL BENEFITS STATEMENT

moregreenmoms saved the following resources by
printing the pages of this book on chlorine free paper
made with 60% post-consumer waste.

TREES	WATER	ENERGY	SOLID WASTE	GREENHOUSE GASES
2	**659**	**1**	**109**	**201**
FULLY GROWN	GALLONS	MILLION BTUs	POUNDS	POUNDS

Calculations based on research by Environmental Defense and the Paper Task Force.
Manufactured at Friesens Corporation

Little Miss Coco **BURST** through the door.

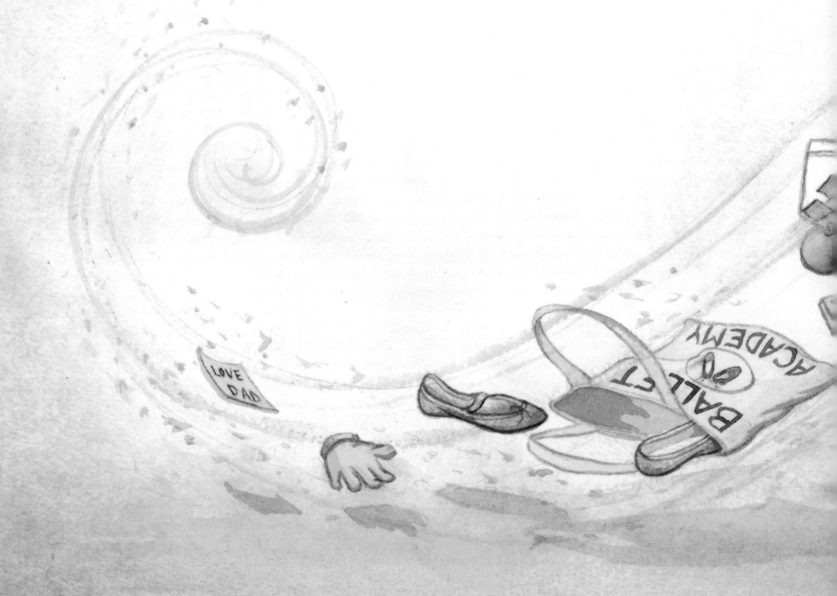

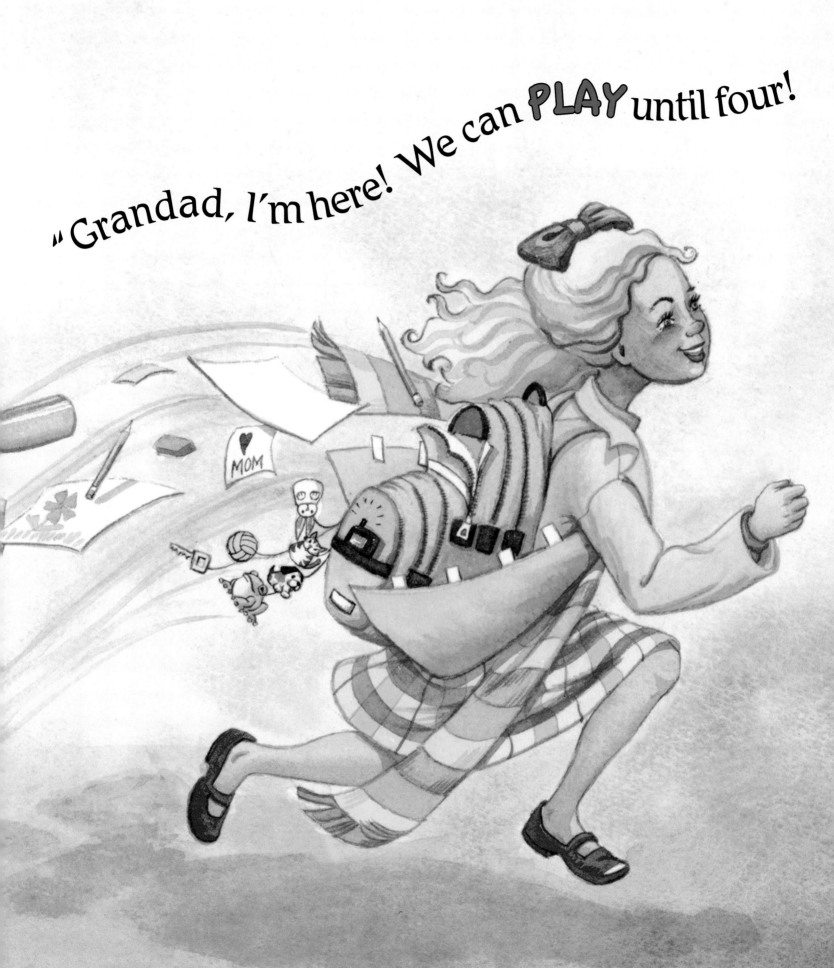

Mommy will **HONK**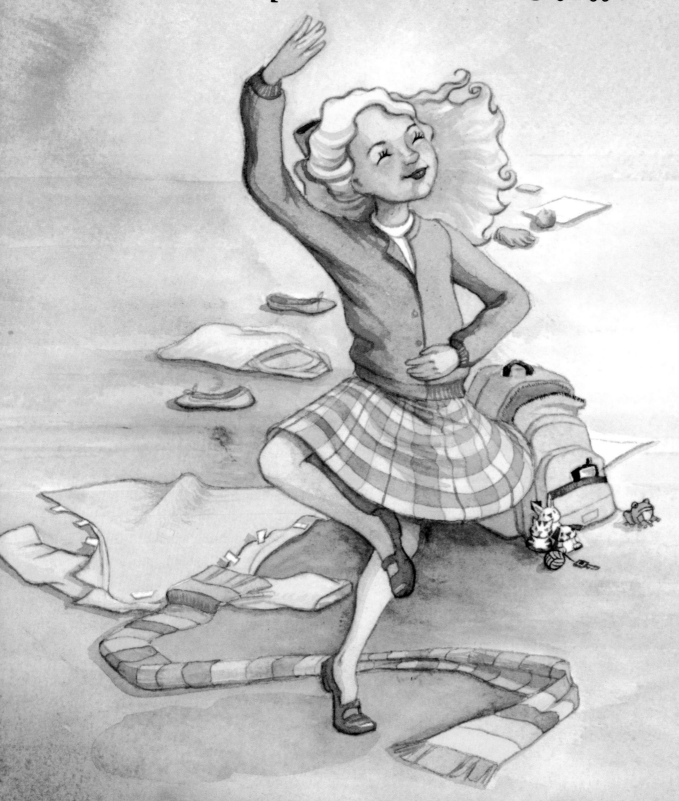

her horn from the car.

Dance class today,

you know I'm the **STAR**."

Grandad just

smiled as she

tipped on her toes.

She makes

a **GRAND**

ENTRANCE

wherever she goes.

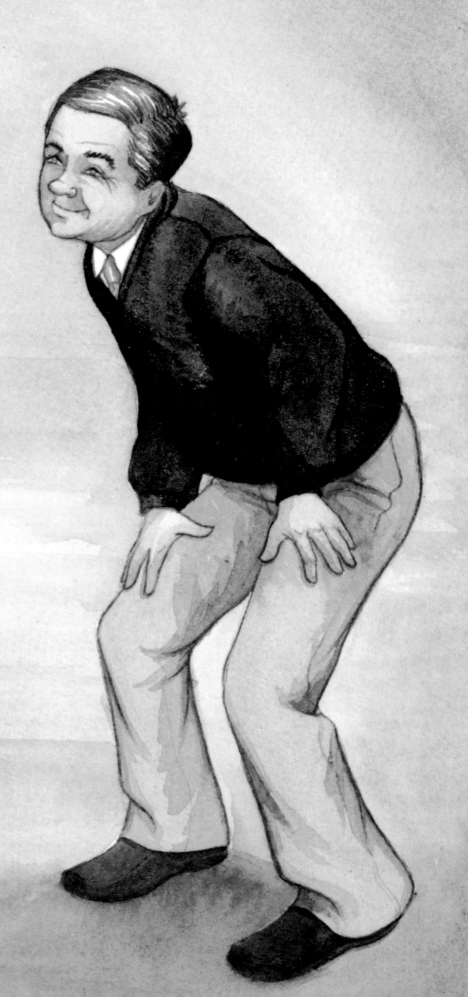

"I ate a great breakfast. I'm ready for you!
Where will we go? What will we do?"

He winked and he TWINKLED
his lovely blue eyes,

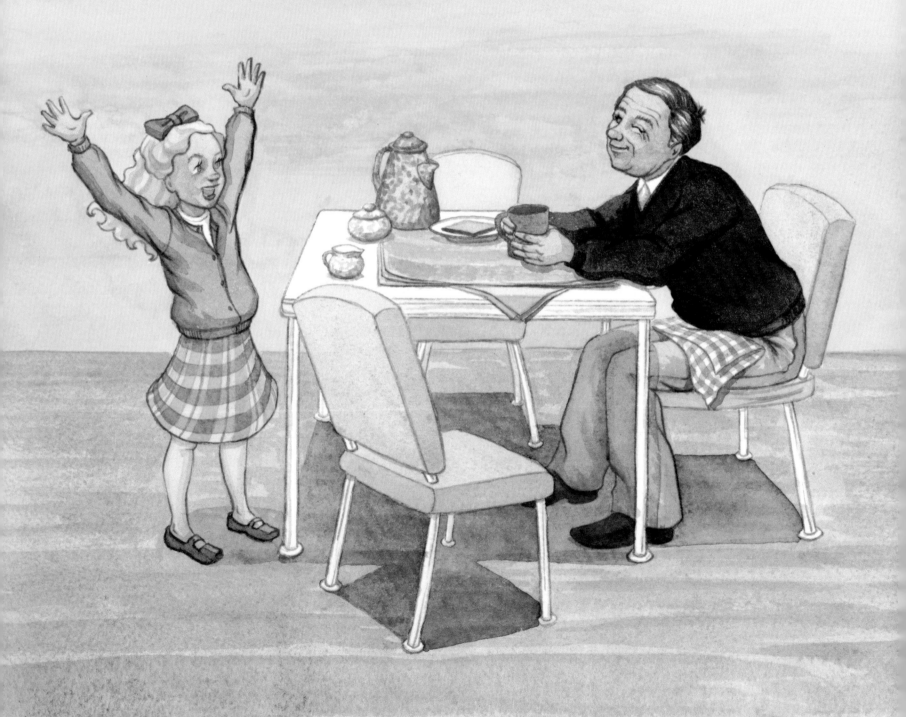

"I thought we'd stay home.
How's THAT for surprise?"

Coco stopped short,
what did he say?

No schedule,

no classes,

no outing today?

Her life is a whirl.
She LOVES to be busy.
Her BLUE RIBBON schedule
does not make her dizzy.

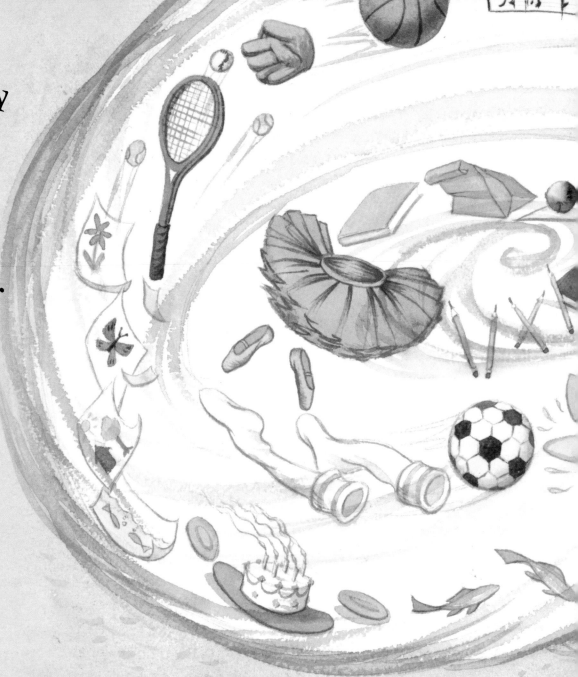

She began as a baby in Mommy and Me and her pace has increased, making time much less free.

Now that she's six, she has school on most days.

But it's the rest of her life that keeps her **ABLAZE**.

Ballet in her tutu, soccer with socks, skating with mittens, art class in smocks, gymnastics for cartwheels, piano for grace, activities and playdates all over the place.

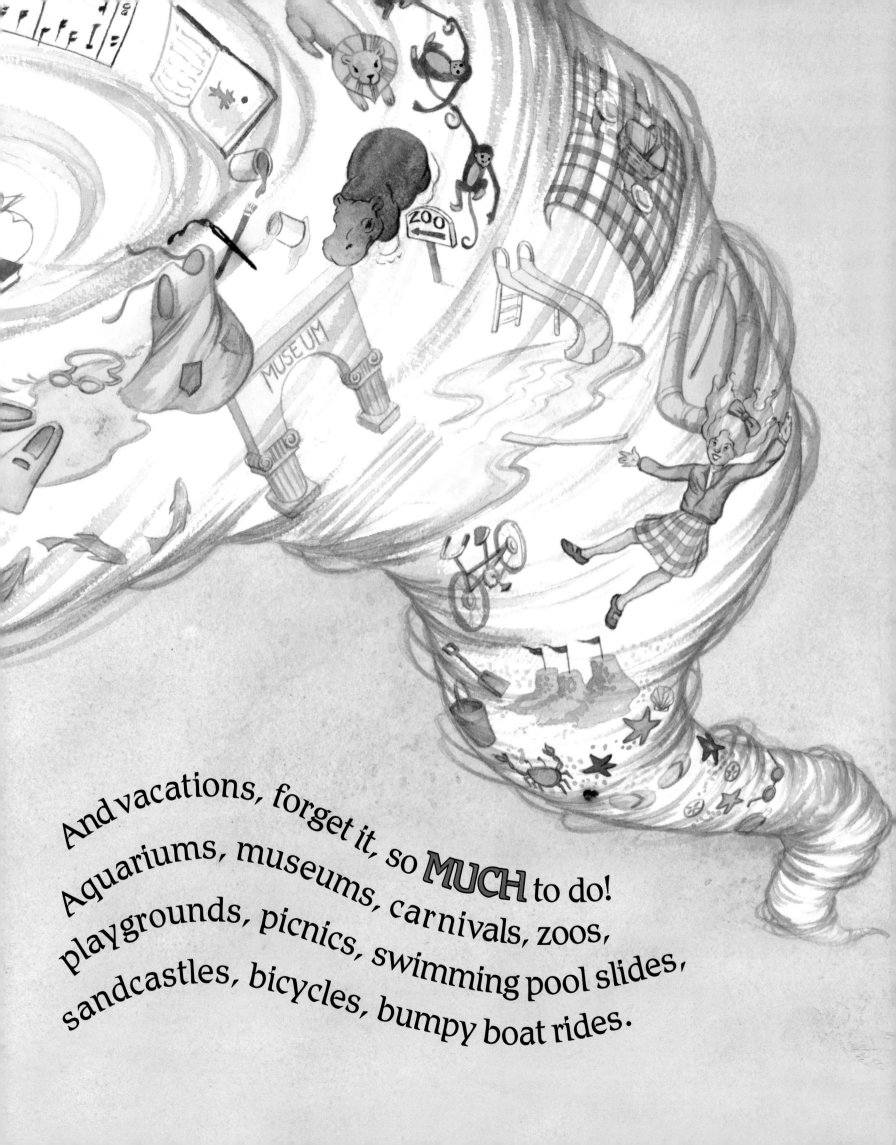

And vacations, forget it, so MUCH to do!
Aquariums, museums, carnivals, zoos,
playgrounds, picnics, swimming pool slides,
sandcastles, bicycles, bumpy boat rides.

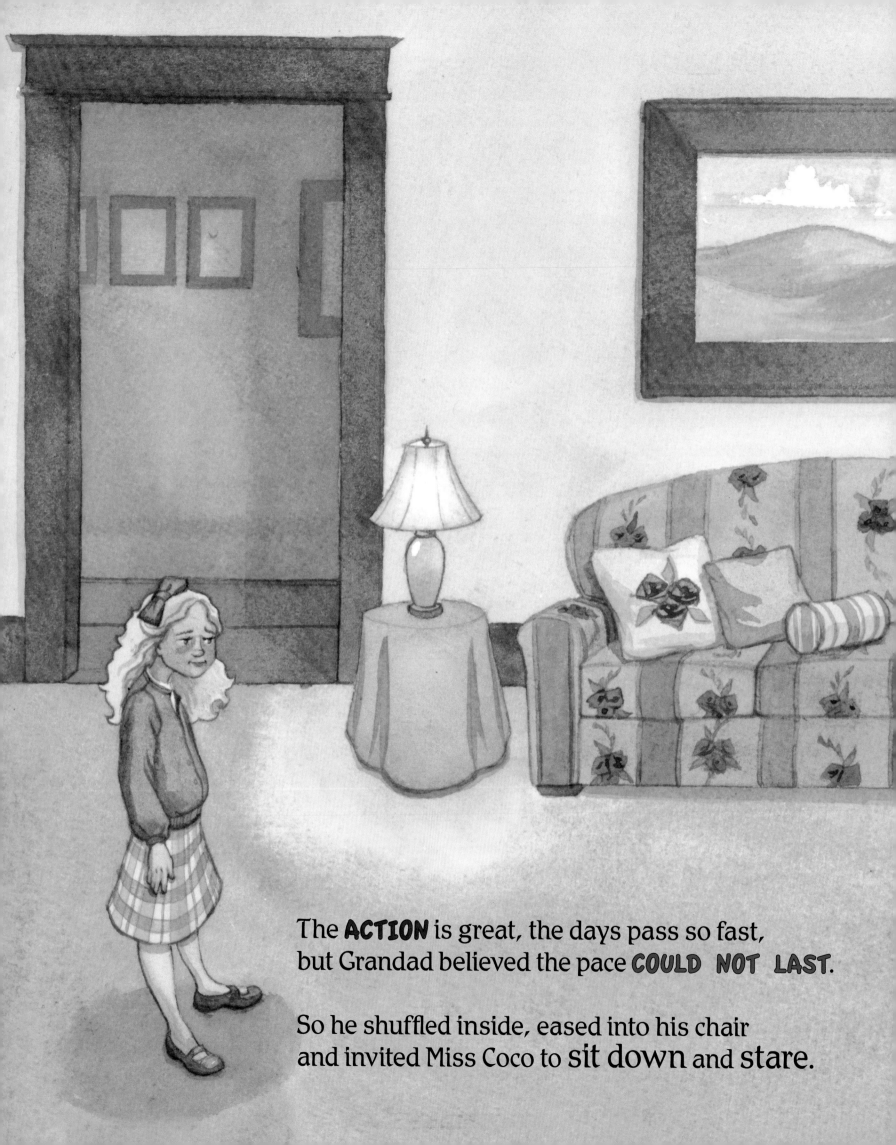

The **ACTION** is great, the days pass so fast,
but Grandad believed the pace COULD NOT LAST.

So he shuffled inside, eased into his chair
and invited Miss Coco to sit down and stare.

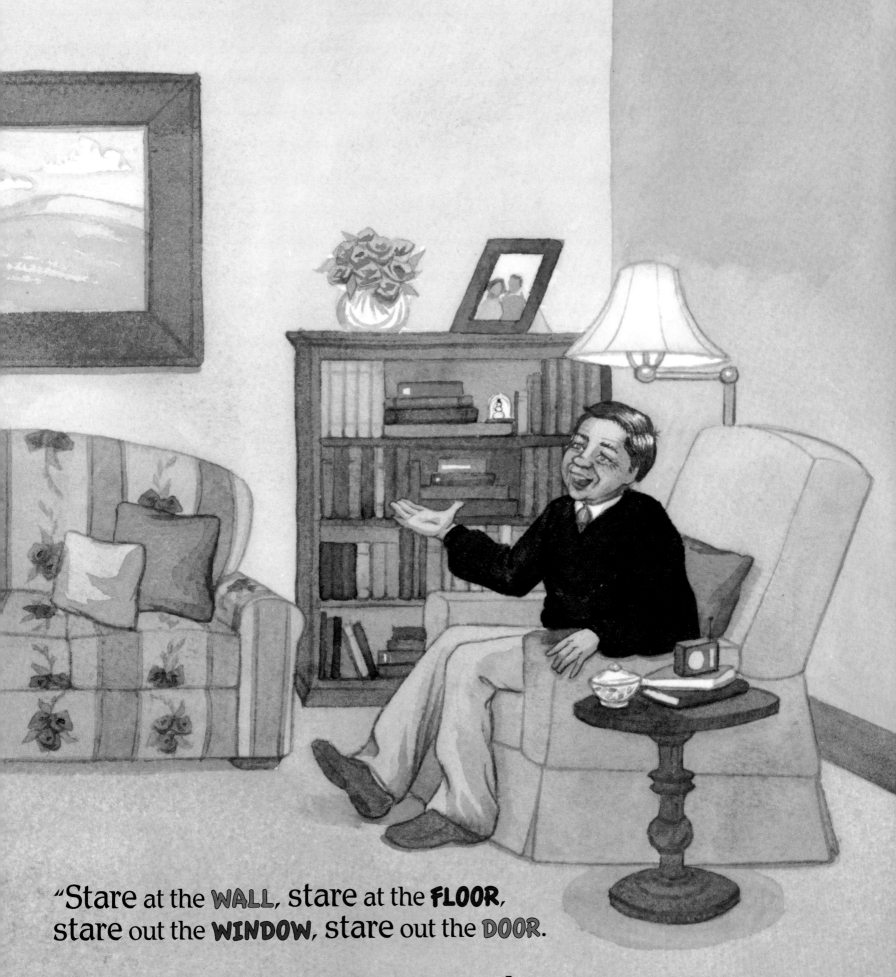

"Stare at the **WALL**, stare at the **FLOOR**,
stare out the **WINDOW**, stare out the **DOOR**.

Let your mind wander, let your breath s l o w.
There's a Coco inside you I want you to know."

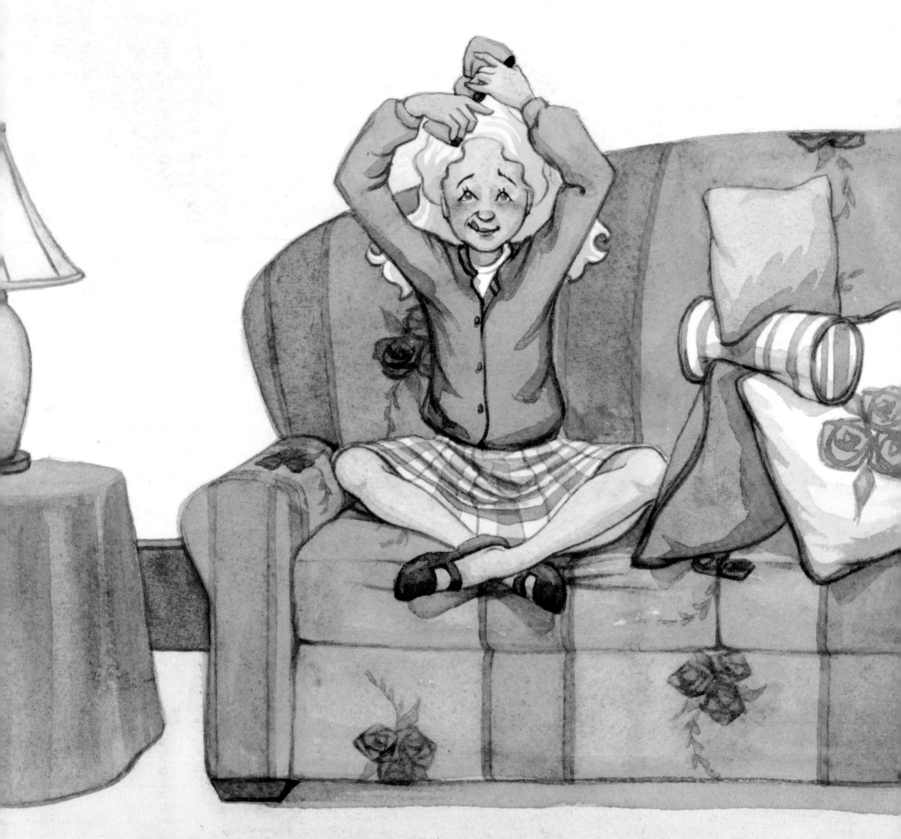

She was **very** confused, but what could she do.
She had to be **quiet** for a moment or two.

She adjusted her bow and scooched on the couch,
fiddled with pillows and tried not to slouch.

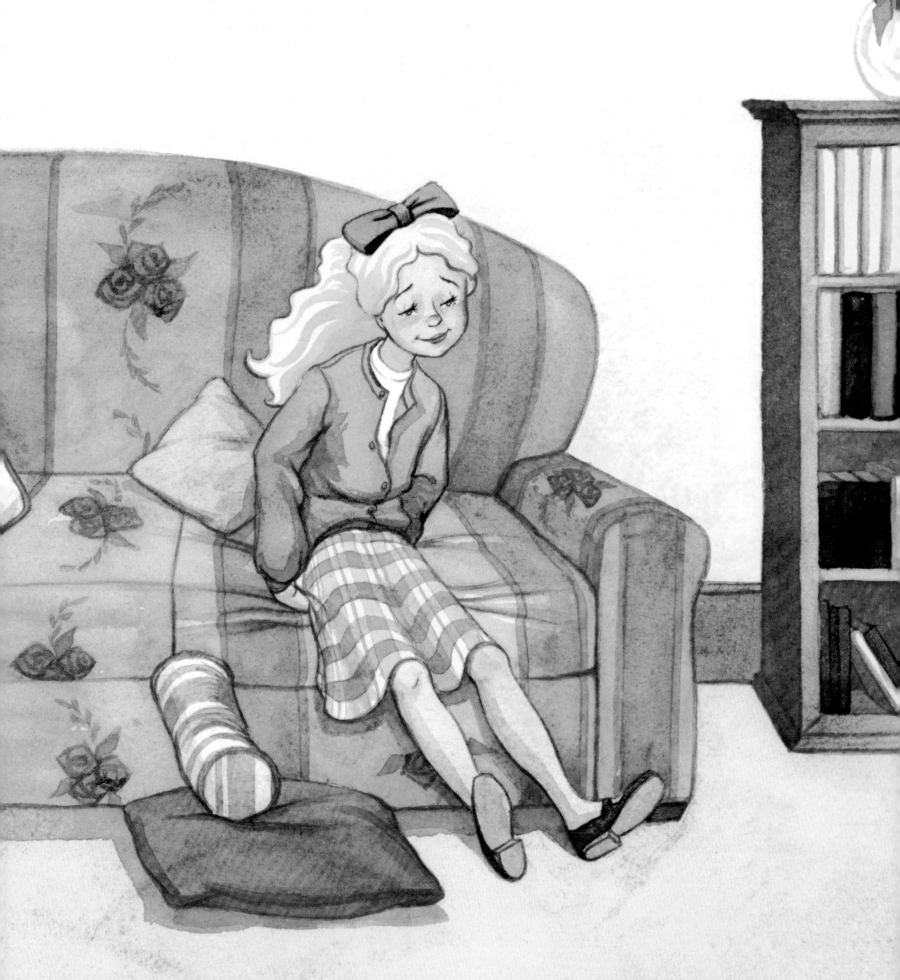

She sat on her hands and admired her shoes,
red MaryJanes, **SHINY** and **NEW**.

She had to think *fast*
to make the time **FLY.**
So she took a DEEP BREATH
and let out a sigh.

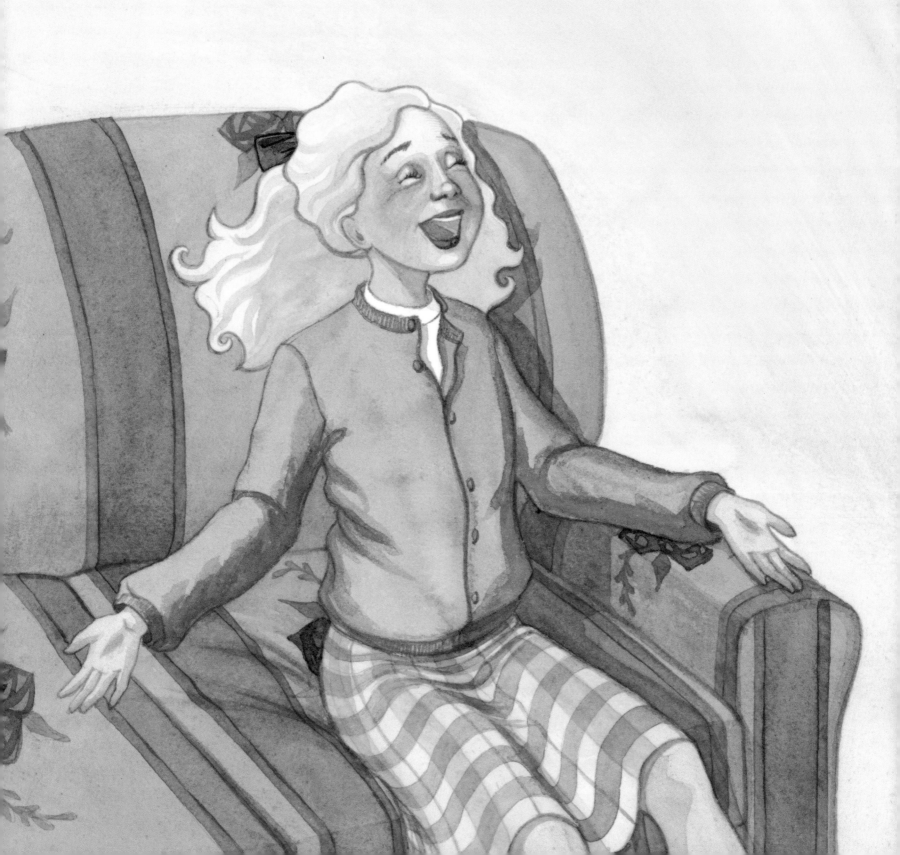

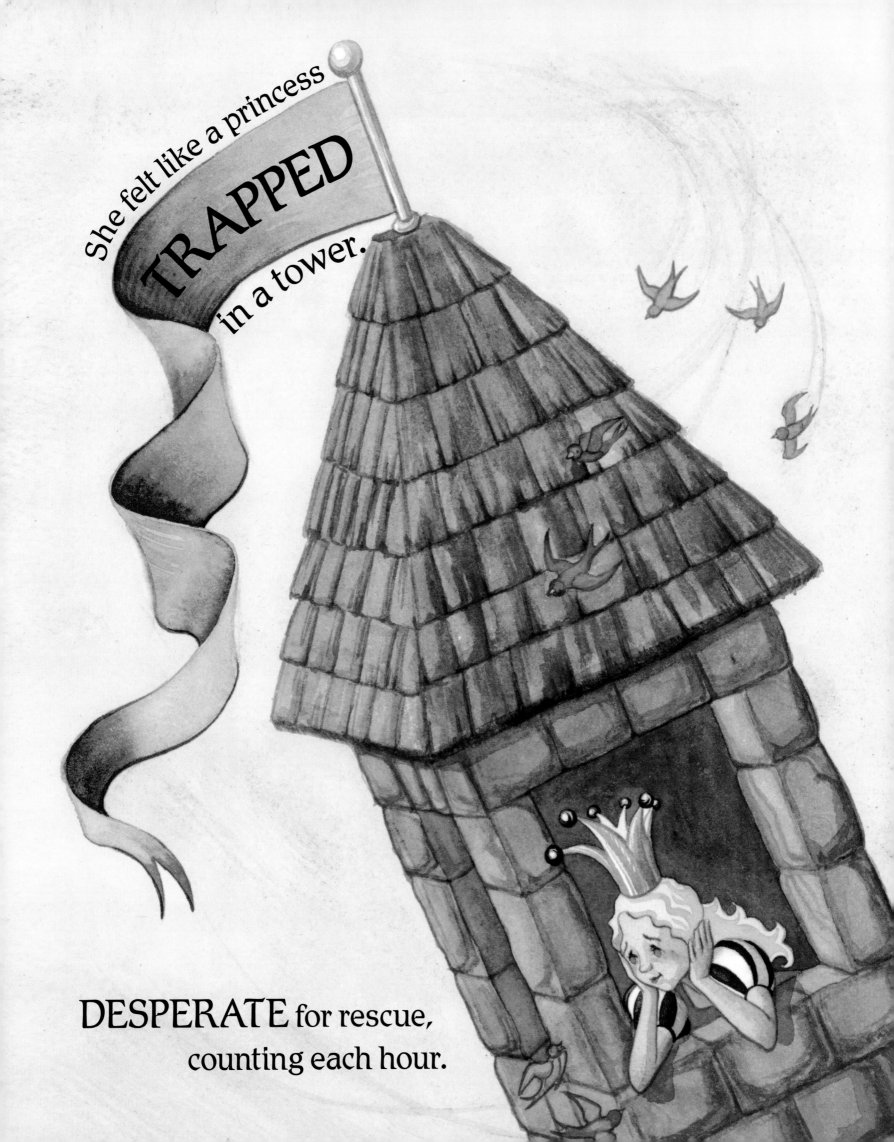

She felt like a princess **TRAPPED** in a tower.

DESPERATE for rescue, counting each hour.

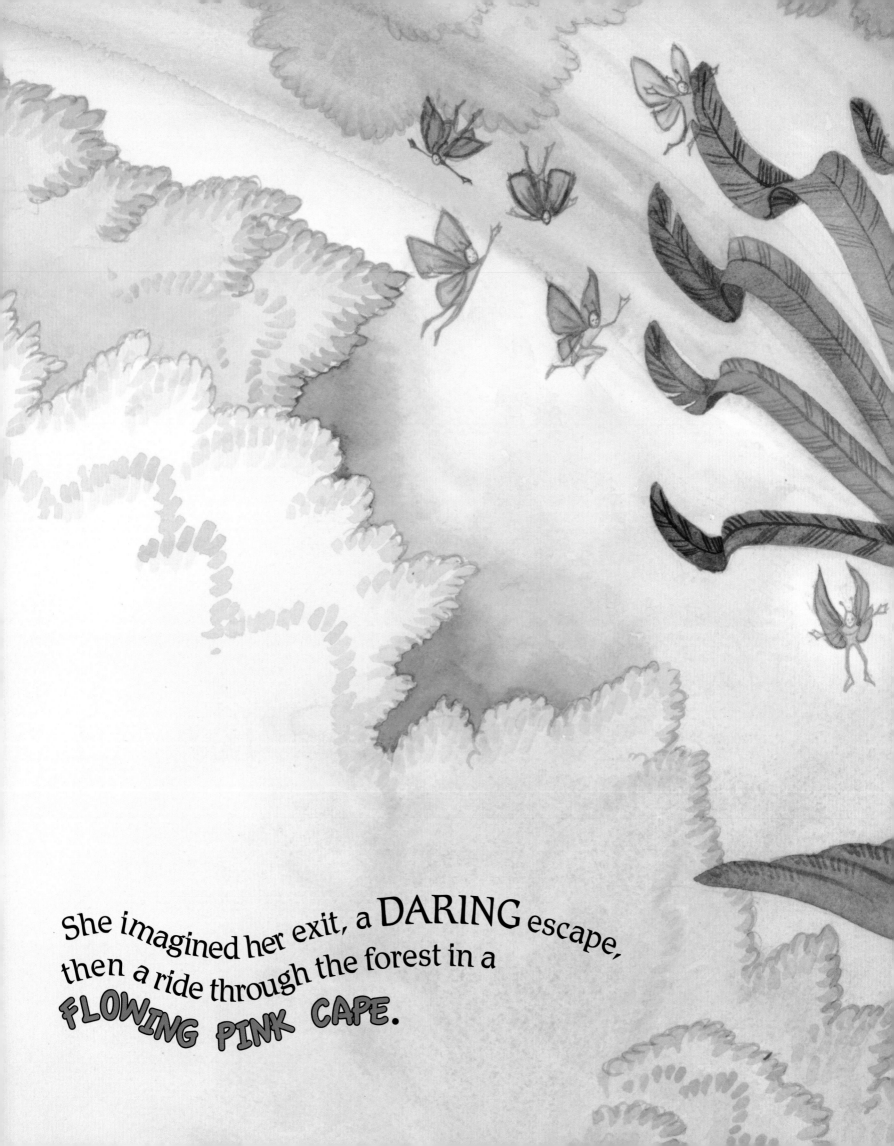

She imagined her exit, a DARING escape, then a ride through the forest in a FLOWING PINK CAPE.

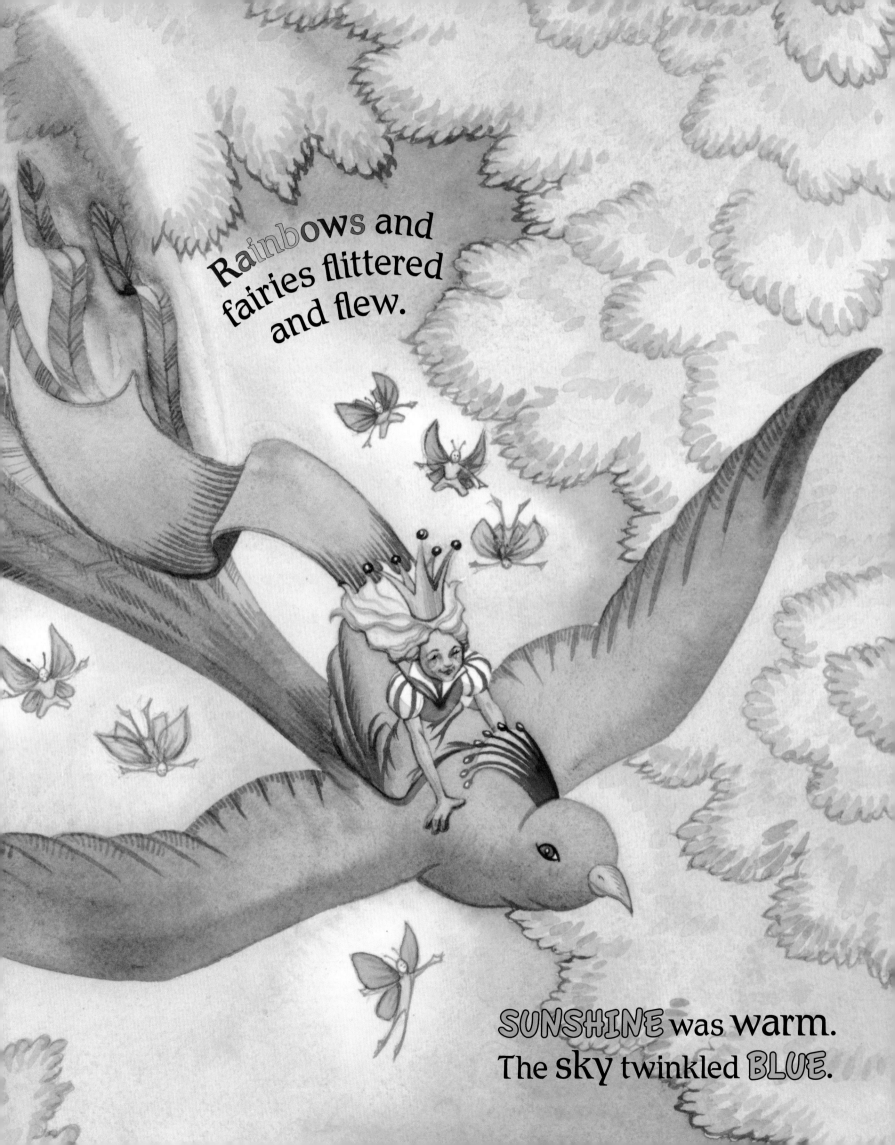

Rainbows and fairies flittered and flew.

SUNSHINE was warm. The sky twinkled BLUE.

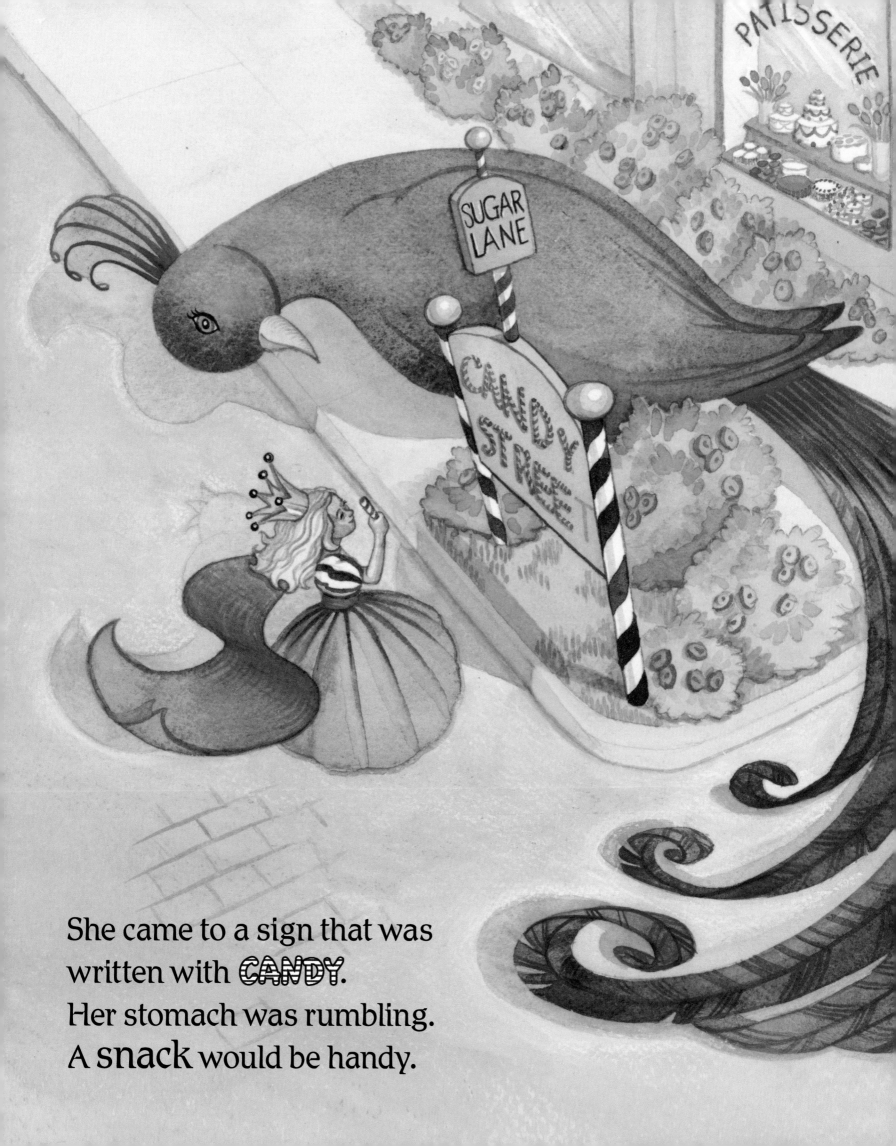

She came to a sign that was
written with CANDY.
Her stomach was rumbling.
A **snack** would be handy.

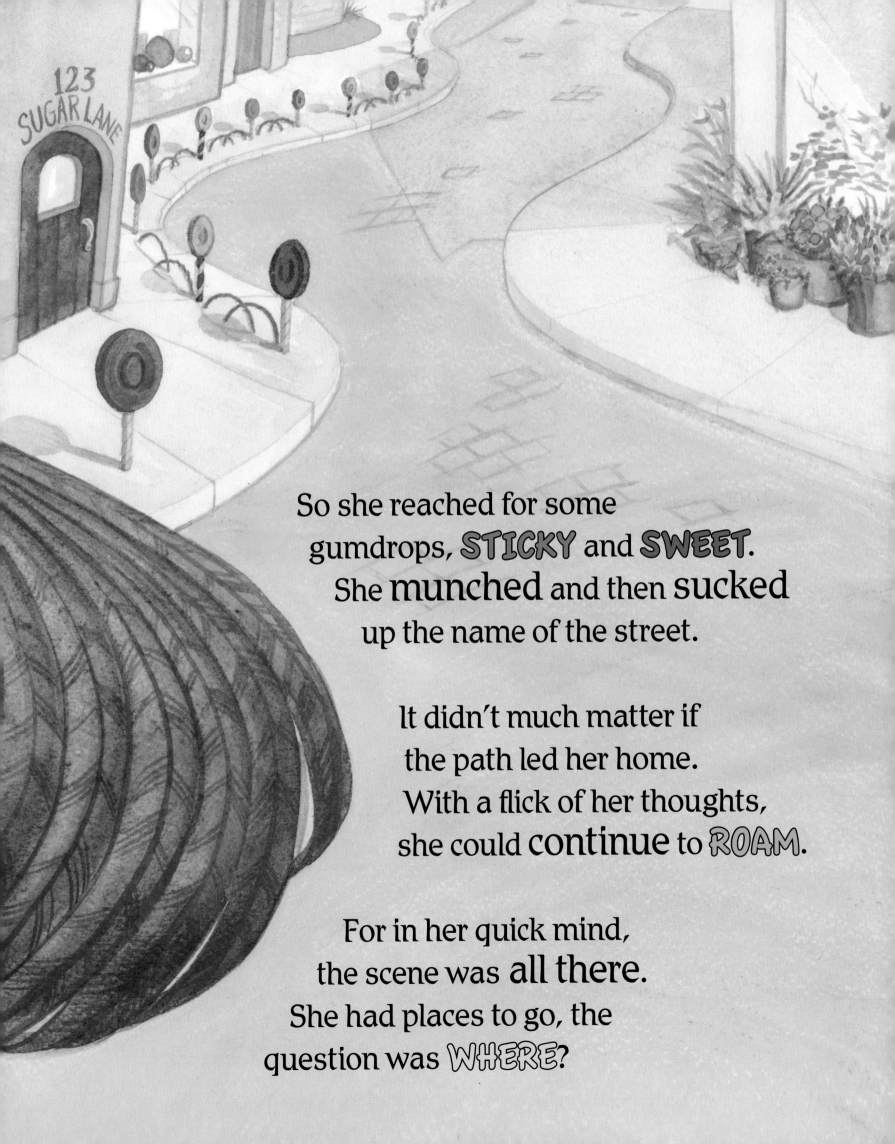

So she reached for some
gumdrops, STICKY and SWEET.
She munched and then sucked
up the name of the street.

It didn't much matter if
the path led her home.
With a flick of her thoughts,
she could continue to ROAM.

For in her quick mind,
the scene was all there.
She had places to go, the
question was WHERE?

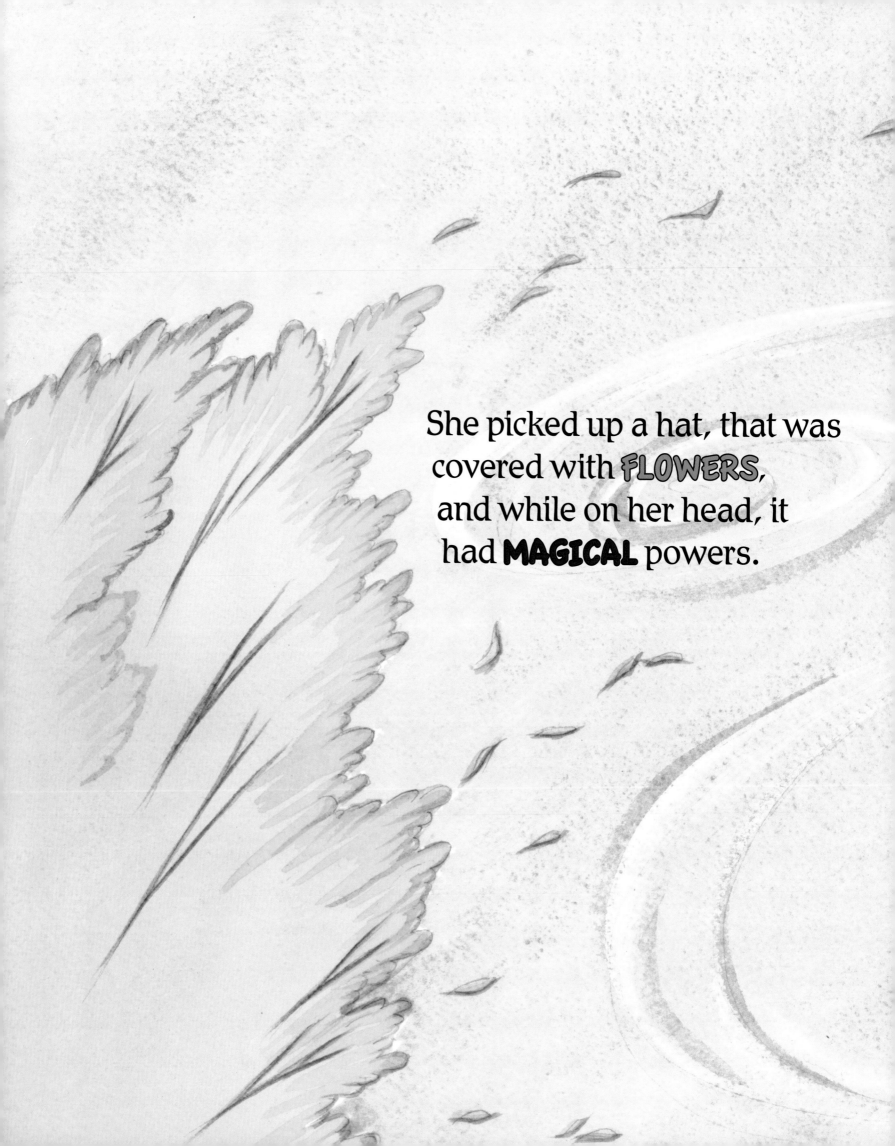

She picked up a hat, that was
covered with FLOWERS,
and while on her head, it
had MAGICAL powers.

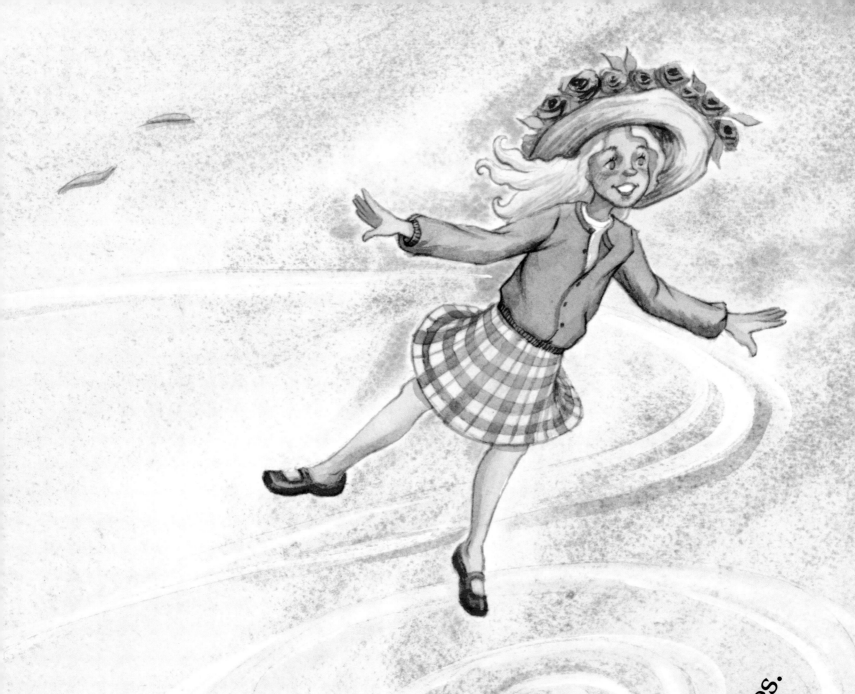

If she tipped the brim left, she could SOAR through the trees.

If she tugged on the right, she could RACE with the breeze.

And when she grew tired of WALKING ON AIR,
she could simply remove it and LAND on a chair.

She would rest there a bit, then GAZE at the sky
and soak in the moon
with a blink of her eye.

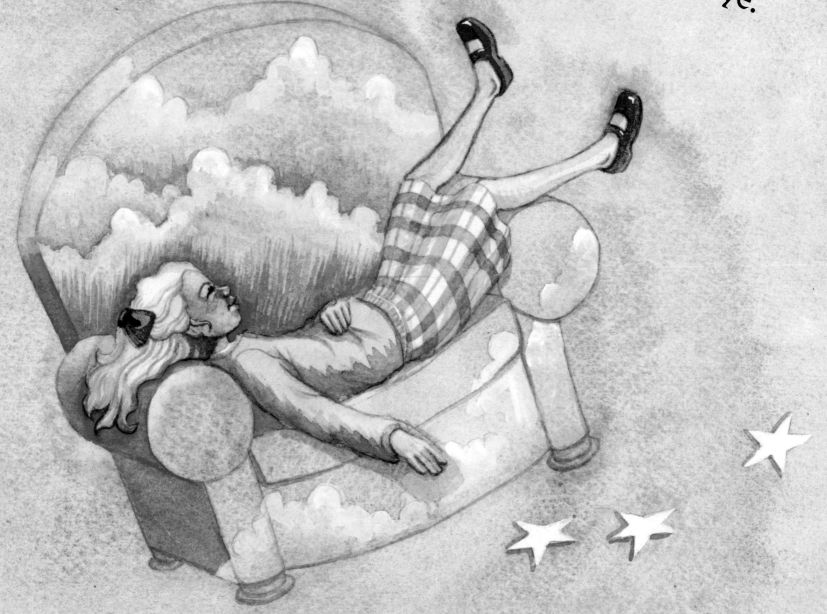

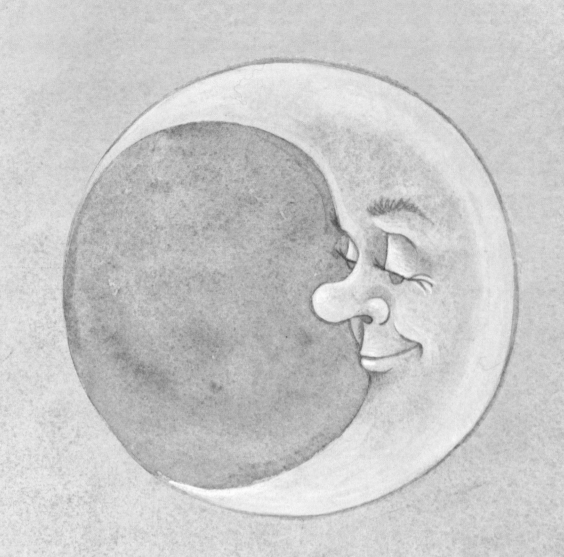

She was **happily** lost in her thoughts of the stars,
wondering if rabbits slurp **ICE CREAM** on Mars,

when her gaze caught a glimpse of Grandad's sweet face,
sleepy and smiley in his most favorite place.

"Hi there," he said. "So tell me, dear one,
did you find in your **QUIET**, a **MOMENT** of **FUN?**"

"Oh, I did," she exclaimed. "I TICKLED the sky

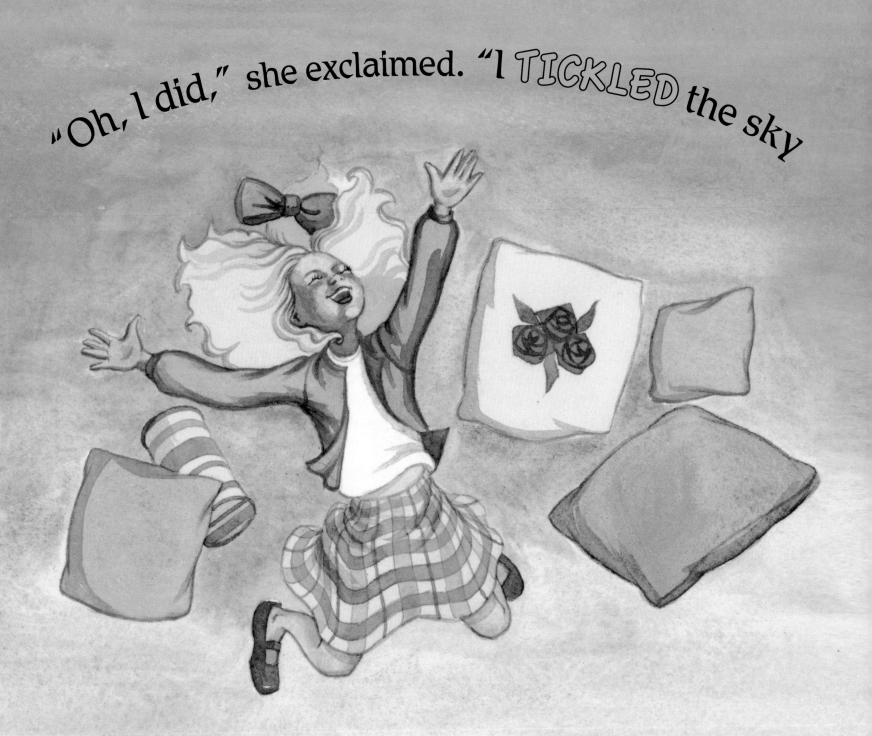

and giggled with sparrows who taught me to FLY.

I took a deep breath, just like you said,
and let the pure magic DANCE in my head."

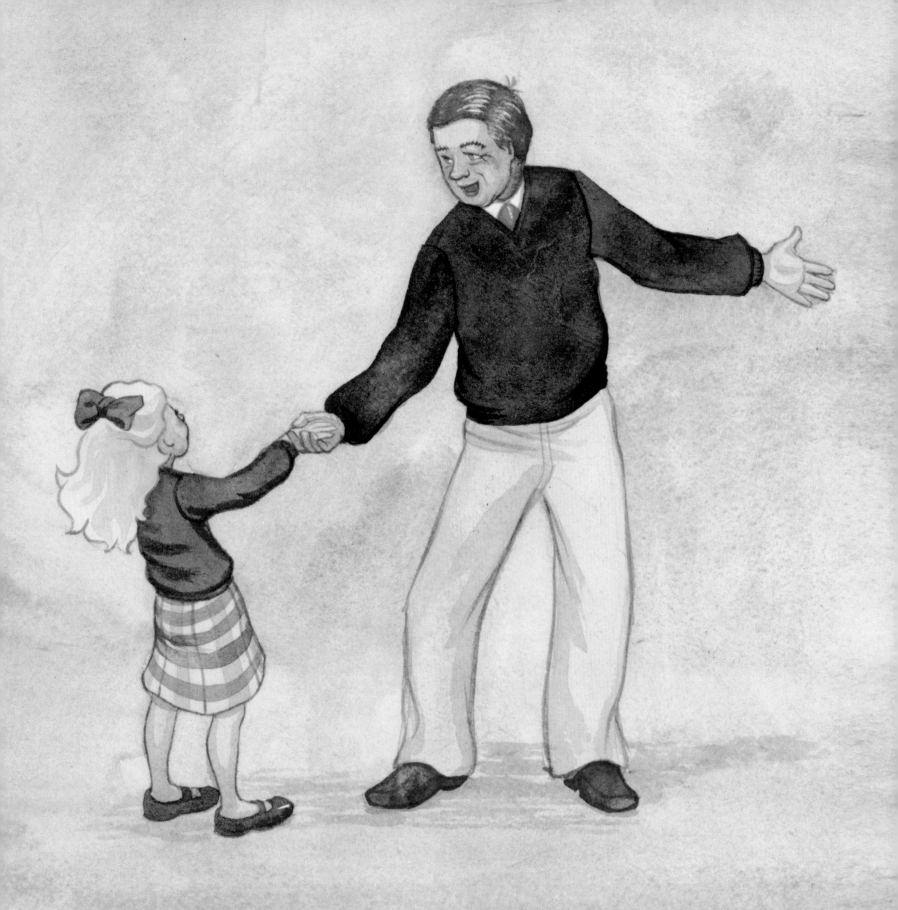

He reached for her **hand** and gave it a **kiss**,
then delivered this message to **dear Little Miss.**

"You can **VOYAGE** clear
out to the **end** of the **sea**.

You can take **all your
friends** or travel with me.

You can wear your
BLUE BOOTS, or
feathers for shoes.

You can come home for dinner
- **or not** - if you choose.

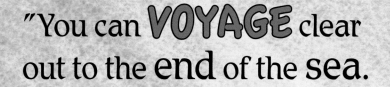

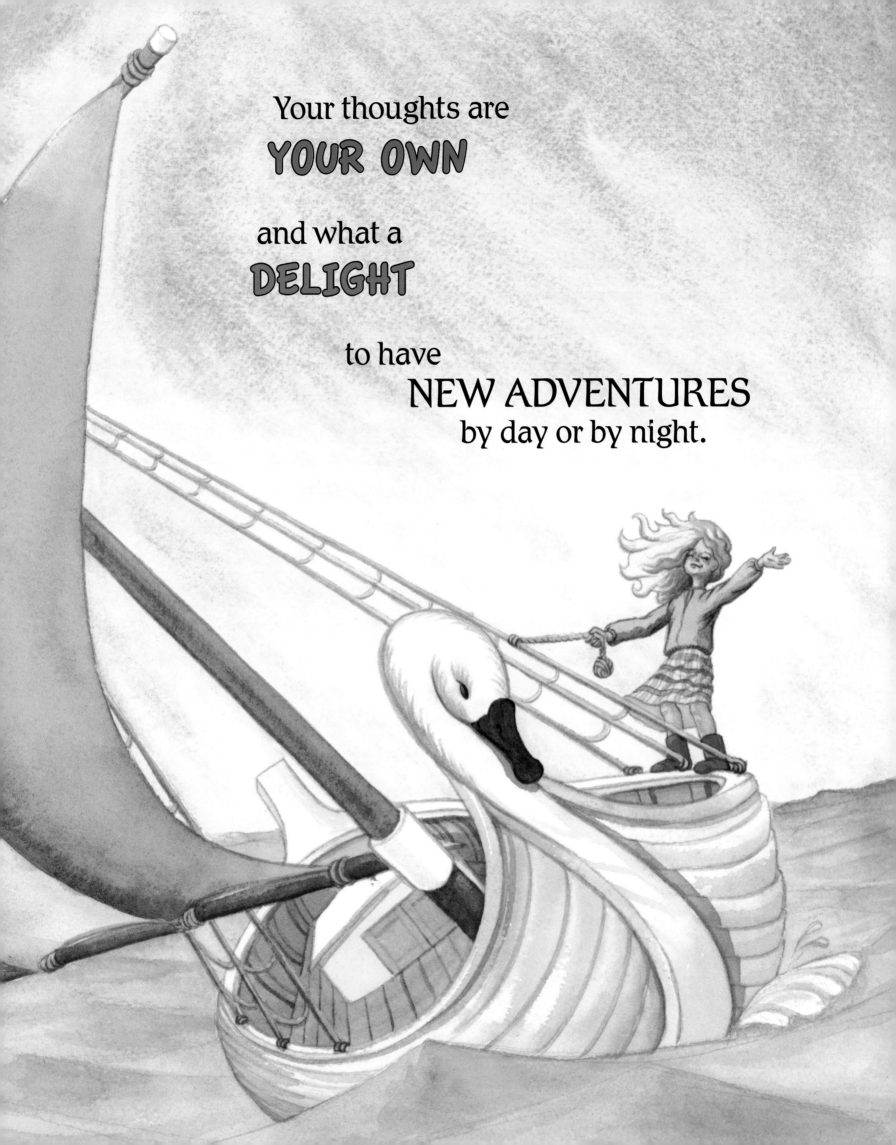

Your thoughts are
YOUR OWN

and what a
DELIGHT

to have
NEW ADVENTURES
by day or by night.

Give yourself **space** and **time** to let go.
This is my treasure, the secret l know.

Life may feel **full** when excitement is near,
But a **MOMENT** of **QUIET** is **NOTHING** to **FEAR**."

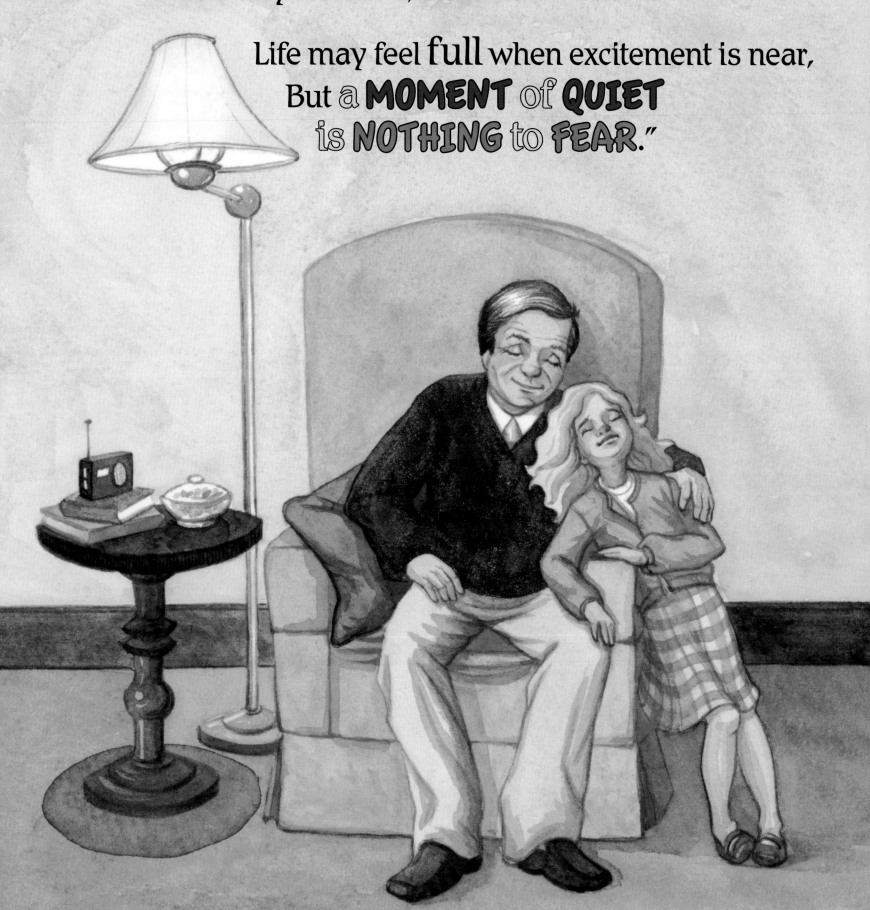